W9-CBH-820

OTHER TITLES OF INTEREST

CODING AND REIMBURSEMENT

Capitation: Tools, Trends, Traps and Techniques
Codelink® Guides to ICD-9-CM and CPT Linkages
Collections Made Easy!
CPT Coders Choice®, Thumb Indexed
CPT & HCPCS Coding Made Easy!
E/M Coding Made Easy!
HCPCS Coders Choice®
Health Insurance Carrier Directory
ICD-9-CM Coders Choice®, Thumb Indexed
ICD-9-CM Coding For Physicians' Offices
ICD-9-CM Coding Made Easy!
Medicare Rules and Regulations
Physicians Fees Guide
Reimbursement Manual for the Medical Office
Working with Insurance and Managed Care Plans

PRACTICE MANAGEMENT

365 Ways to Manage the Business Called Private Practice
Achieving Profitability with a Medical Office System
Behavioral Types and the Art of Patient Management
Computerizing Your Medical Office
Doctor Business
Encyclopedia of Practice and Financial Management
Getting Paid for What You Do
Health Information Management
Managed Care Handbook
Managing Medical Office Personnel
McGraw-Hill Pocket Guide to Managed Care
Medical Marketing Handbook
Medical Practice Handbook
Medical Staff Privileges
Negotiating Managed Care Contracts
New Practice Handbook
Patient Satisfaction
Patients Build Your Practice
Physician's Office Laboratory
Professional and Practice Development
Promoting Your Medical Practice
Starting in Medical Practice

AVAILABLE FROM YOUR LOCAL MEDICAL BOOK STORE OR CALL 1-800-MED-SHOP

OTHER TITLES OF INTEREST

FINANCIAL MANAGEMENT

Accounts Receivable Management for Medical Practice
Business Ventures for Physicians
Financial Planning Workbook for Physicians
Financial Valuation of Your Practice
Pension Plan Strategies
Physician Financial Planning in a Changing Environment
Securing Your Assets
Selling or Buying a Medical Practice

RISK MANAGEMENT

Malpractice Depositions
Malpractice: Managing Your Defense
Testifying in Court

DICTIONARIES AND OTHER REFERENCE

Medical Acronyms, Eponyms and Abbreviations
Medical Phrase Index
Medical Word Building
Medico-Legal Glossary
Medico Mnemonica
Spanish/English Handbook for Medical Professionals

MEDICAL REFERENCE AND CLINICAL

Anesthesiology: Problems in Primary Care
Cardiology: Problems in Primary Care
Drugs of Abuse
Gastroenterology: Problems in Primary Care
Medical Care of the Adolescent Athlete
Medical Procedures for Referral
Neurology: Problems in Primary Care
Orthopaedics: Problems in Primary Care
Patient Care Emergency Handbook
Patient Care Flowchart Manual
Patient Care Procedures for Your Practice
Questions and Answers on AIDS
Sexually Transmitted Diseases
Urology: Problems in Primary Care

AVAILABLE FROM YOUR LOCAL MEDICAL BOOK STORE OR CALL 1-800-MED-SHOP

ICD·9·CM

CODING MADE EASY!

A Comprehensive Coding Guide for Health Care Professionals

Second Edition

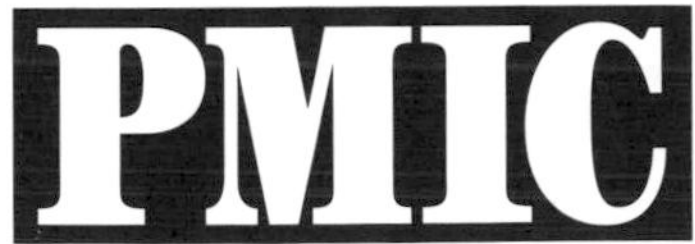

Davis, James B. and Stone, Beverly J.

ISBN 1-57066-184-7

Practice Management Information Corporation (PMIC)
4727 Wilshire Blvd.
Los Angeles, California 90010
1-800-MED-SHOP
http://www.medicalbookstore.com

Printed in the United States of America

Copyright© 2000 under the Uniform Copyright Convention. All rights reserved. This book is protected by copyright. No part of it may be reproduced, stored in a retrieval system, or transmitted in any form or by any means, electronic, mechanical, photocopying, recording, or otherwise, without written permission from the publisher.

PREFACE

ICD-9-CM Coding Made Easy! is a comprehensive coding guide designed specifically for use with the International Classification of Diseases, 9th Revision, Clinical Modification, commonly known as ICD-9-CM. It is intended as an introduction to the ICD-9-CM coding system and the Medicare ICD-9-CM coding rules and regulations.

Health care professionals have long used coding systems to describe procedures, services, and supplies. However, most described the reason for the procedure, service or supply with a diagnostic statement. Of those health care professionals who do code the diagnosis, either due to a requirement for a computer billing system and/or electronic claims filing, many do not code completely or accurately. With the passage of the Medicare Catastrophic Coverage Act of 1988, diagnostic coding using ICD-9-CM became mandatory for Medicare claims. In the area of health care reimbursement rules and regulations, the typical progression is that changes required for Medicare are followed shortly by similar changes for Medicaid and private insurance carriers.

To some professionals, the requirement to use diagnostic coding may seem a burden or simply another excuse for Medicare intermediaries to delay or deny payment. However, it is important to understand that the proper use of coding systems for both procedures and diagnoses gives the professional absolute control over his or her billing and reimbursement. Accurate diagnosis coding is not easy. It requires a good working knowledge of medical terminology and a fundamental understanding of ICD-9-CM. In addition, the coder must know the rules and regulations required to comply with Medicare requirements for coding.

ICD-9-CM Coding Made Easy! provides the information necessary to develop a fundamental understanding of ICD-9-CM coding as well as the steps needed to comply fully with the new Medicare rules and regulations governing ICD-9-CM coding.

DISCLAIMER

This publication is designed to offer basic information regarding the proper use of ICD-9-CM coding and to provide a reliable source of understanding Medicare regulations regarding ICD-9-CM. The information regarding coding and billing is based on the experience and interpretations of the authors. Though all the information has been checked for accuracy and completeness, neither the authors nor the publisher accept any responsibility or liability with regard to errors, omissions, misuse or misinterpretation.

THE AUTHORS

JAMES B. DAVIS

James B. Davis has been in the health care field for over 25 years working closely with medical professionals, hospitals and insurance carriers. He founded one of California's most successful medical billing companies in 1978. In 1986 he founded PMIC, which has become the nation's number one publisher and distributor of practice management and reimbursement books. He is the author, editor or publisher of many other practice management publications.

BEVERLY J. STONE

Beverly J. Stone has been working with health care professionals for many years. A popular speaker, she has given numerous seminars on the subjects of CPT and ICD-9-CM coding to health care professionals. Ms. Stone is the founder and President of Provider Billing Services, a California based medical billing firm.

CONTENTS

CONTENTS

CONTENTS

CONTENTS

INTRODUCTION

This section deals with some of the most significant reimbursement issues associated with diagnosis coding. You will learn the basic steps of preparing your practice for ICD-9-CM coding and all of the Medicare rules and regulations which require this coding system.

Prior to the Medicare Catastrophic Coverage Act of 1988 (subsequently repealed), most medical professionals used diagnosis text on insurance claims. Instead of putting a diagnosis code on an insurance claim form, they simply wrote the diagnosis, complaint, injury or symptoms. Diagnosis coding was already prevalent in hospital medical record departments; however, other medical professionals used ICD-9-CM codes only if they were computerized. As of this revision of this tutorial, most medical professionals now use ICD-9-CM coding to some degree.

PREPARING FOR ICD-9-CM CODING

Proper preparation for converting your practice to ICD-9-CM coding is a four-step process. The four steps include evaluating your coding resources, reviewing your diagnostic statements, training and development, and preparing an ICD-9 master list for your practice.
Even if your practice is already using ICD-9-CM coding you will need to review the following steps and take appropriate action where necessary.

EVALUATE YOUR RESOURCES

Coding Materials

- Do you have a current copy of *ICD-9-CM, Fourth Edition*?
- Do you have a copy for each person involved in the coding and billing process?
- Are you still using outdated editions of ICD-9-CM?

Coding Expertise

- Do you have staff with sufficient coding expertise to prepare your practice for ICD-9-CM coding?
- Does the expert coder have enough time to develop and manage the ICD-9-CM coding process?

REVIEW DIAGNOSTIC STATEMENTS

Diagnostic Statements

- Are your diagnostic statements in the medical records accurate and precise?
- Are they easy to read?
- Do you use a lot of "rule out" diagnostic statements?

Superbill

- Are you using a fee ticket or superbill to record your charges and diagnoses?
- If yes, does the superbill have ICD-9-CM codes in addition to written descriptions?
- Are the ICD-9 codes current, accurate and complete?
- Do you have the ability to code fifth digits where required?
- Is there a place on the superbill to relate the diagnosis code to a specific procedure?

TRAINING AND DEVELOPMENT

Purchase Materials

Following completion of the steps outlined above, prepare your practice for ICD-9-CM coding by purchasing necessary materials, such as the *ICD-9-CM, Fifth Edition*, additional copies of ICD-9-CM, or copies of the Official Addenda.

Train Yourself and Staff

If the review reveals a lack of staff coding expertise, plan to send the person(s) designated to manage the practice's ICD-9-CM coding process to seminars for training. We strongly recommend that the health care professional also attend a coding seminar if not well-trained in the area of diagnostic coding.

Supplement the Staff

If the review reveals staff expertise, but lack of staff time, consider hiring additional full or part-time staff to perform the coding function, or to perform the functions of the practice's designated coder. Consider hiring someone from your hospital medical records department.

Improve Your Diagnostic Statements

If the coding review reveals problems with illegible or difficult to read coding statements, excessive use of "rule out" statements, imprecise or inaccurate coding statements, try to improve your efforts in these areas. Keep in mind that this not only makes coding easier for the staff, but it directly affects the practice's reimbursement.

Correct Defiencies in Your Superbill

Redesign your superbill to provide the ability to use ICD-9-CM codes properly, including fifth-digits where required, plus a means to relate the diagnoses specifically to the procedures, services, and/or supplies provided. Make sure you include the ability to write-in and code diagnoses which are not listed.

CREATE AN ICD-9-CM MASTER LIST

Prepare a list of the 50 to 100 diagnoses most frequently used by your practice. Make sure to include appropriate symptoms, signs and other conditions. Indicate the need for fifth digits by using a blank, box, or asterisk next to appropriate codes. Use this list to redesign your superbill or fee ticket. Make sure the health care professional and all staff involved with the coding and billing process are familiar with the list. Review your superbills from time-to-time to determine if you are writing in a lot of unlisted diagnoses. Add these codes to your ICD-9-CM codes master list if they are being used frequently.

MEDICARE REQUIREMENTS FOR ICD-9-CM CODING

The Medicare Catastrophic Coverage Act of 1988 (PL 100-330) requires that health care professionals submit an appropriate diagnosis code, using the International Classification of Diseases, 9th Revision, Clinical Modification (ICD-9-CM) for each procedure, service, or supply billed under Medicare Part B.

To comply with the regulations, health care professionals must convert the reason(s) the procedures, services or supplies were performed or issued, from written diagnostic statements which may include specific diagnoses, signs, symptoms and/or complaints, into ICD-9-CM diagnosis codes. The Health Care Financing Administration originally set the implementation date for this requirement as April 1, 1989; however, it was subsequently delayed until June 1, 1989, at the request of the American Medical Association, to give health care providers additional time to prepare for the change.

HCFA GUIDELINES FOR USING ICD-9-CM CODES

The Health Care Financing Administration (HCFA) has prepared guidelines for using ICD-9-CM codes and instructions on how to report them on claim forms. In addition, HCFA has directed your Medicare intermediary to provide you with a written copy of these instructions. The basic HCFA guidelines are summarized below, however, it is very important that you obtain a copy of the guidelines from your Medicare intermediary as implementation of HCFA requirements varies from one intermediary to another.

1. Indicate on the claim form or itemized statement the appropriate code(s) from the ICD-9-CM code range 001.0 through V82.9 to identify diagnoses, symptoms, conditions, problems, complaints or other reason(s) for the procedure, service or supply provided.

   A. In choosing codes to describe the reason for the encounter, the health care professional will frequently be using codes within the range from 001.0 through 999.9, the section of ICD-9-CM for the classification of diseases and injuries (e.g. infectious and parasitic diseases; neoplasms; signs, symptoms and ill-defined conditions). Codes that describe symptoms as opposed to diagnoses are acceptable if this is the highest level of certainty documented by the physician.

   B. ICD-9-CM also provides codes to deal with visits for circumstances other than a disease or injury, such as an encounter for a laboratory test only. These codes are found in the V-code section and range from V01.0 through V82.9.

2. The ICD-9-CM code for the diagnosis, condition, problem, or other reason for the encounter documented in the medical record as the main reason for the procedure, service or supply provided should be listed first. Additional ICD-9-CM codes that describe any current coexisting conditions are then listed. Do not include codes for conditions that were previously treated and no longer exist.

3. ICD-9-CM codes should be used at their highest level of specificity.

   A. Assign three digit codes only if there are no four digit codes within the coding category.

   B. Assign four digit codes only if there is no fifth digit subclassification for that category.

   C. Assign the fifth digit subclassification code for those categories where it exists.

Claims submitted with three or four digit codes where four and five digit codes are available may be returned to you by the Medicare intermediary for proper coding. It is recognized that a very specific diagnosis may not be known at the time of the initial encounter. However, that is not an acceptable reason to submit a three digit code when four or five digits are available.

For example, if the patient has chronic bronchitis, ICD-9-CM code 491, and the physician has not yet documented whether the bronchitis is simple, mucopurulent, or obstructive, the code for unspecified chronic bronchitis, ICD-9-CM code 491.9, should be listed.

4. Diagnoses documented as "probable," "suspected," "questionable," or "rule out" should not be coded as if the diagnosis is confirmed. The condition(s) should be coded to the highest degree of certainty for the encounter, such as describing symptoms, signs, abnormal test results, or other reasons for the encounter.

5. Chronic disease(s) treated on an ongoing basis may be coded and reported as many times as the patient receives treatment and care for the condition(s).

6. When patients receive ancillary diagnostic services only during an encounter, the appropriate "V code" for the service should be listed first, and the diagnosis or problem for which the diagnostic procedures are being performed should be listed second.

   A. V codes will be used frequently by radiologists who perform radiological examinations on referrals. For example, ICD-9-CM code V72.5, Radiological examination, not elsewhere classified, describes the reason for the encounter and should be listed first on the claim form or statement. If the reason for the referral is known, a second ICD-9-CM code which describes the signs or symptoms for which the examination was ordered should be listed.

   B. Failure to list a second ICD-9-CM code in addition to the V code may result in claim delays or denials. The ICD-9-CM code V72.5, Radiological examination, not elsewhere classified, includes referrals for routine chest x-rays that are not covered by the Medicare program. Medicare intermediaries may establish screening programs to verify that the referrals were not for routine chest x-rays.

By supplying a second ICD-9-CM code to describe the reason for the referral, these claims can be clearly identified by the Medicare intermediary as referrals to evaluate symptoms, signs or diagnoses. The mission of a second ICD-9-CM code may lead to requests for additional information from Medicare intermediaries prior to processing the claim.

7. For patients receiving only ancillary therapeutic services during an encounter, list the appropriate V code first, followed by the ICD-9-CM code for the diagnosis or problem for which the services are being performed. For example, a patient with multiple sclerosis presenting for rehabilitation services would be coded using code V57.1, Other physical therapy, or code V57.89, Other specified rehabilitation procedure, followed by code 340, Multiple sclerosis.

8. For surgical procedures, use the ICD-9-CM code for the diagnosis for which the surgery was performed. If the postoperative diagnosis is known to be different at the time the claim is filed, use the ICD-9-CM code for the postoperative diagnosis.

9. Code all documented conditions that coexist at the time of the visit that require or affect patient care, treatment or management. Do not code conditions that were previously treated and no longer exist.

COMPLETING THE HCFA1500 CLAIM FORM

Health care professionals using the Uniform Health Insurance Claim Form, HCFA1500, to file claims for services provided to Medicare beneficiaries must list a minimum of one ICD-9-CM code and may list up to four ICD-9-CM codes on the claim form.

The ICD-9-CM code for the diagnosis, condition, problem or other reason for the encounter is listed first, followed by up to three additional codes that describe any coexisting conditions. At times, there may be several conditions that equally resulted in the encounter. In these cases, the health care professional is free to select the one that will be listed first.

The ICD-9-CM codes are listed in Box 21 of the HCFA1500 claim form (see example). In addition, in Box 24 D of the form, you must indicate by a number from 1 to 4, or combination of numbers, which diagnoses from Box 21 support the procedure, service or supply listed in Box 24 C.

Due to space limitations on the claim form you may use only up to four ICD-9-CM codes for diagnoses, conditions, or signs and symptoms. Frequently the patient may have more than four conditions present at the time of the encounter, however, you must choose only four codes to be listed on the claim form.

21. DIAGNOSIS OR NATURE OF ILLNESS OR INJURY. (RELATE ITEMS 1,2,3 OR 4 TO ITEM 24E BY LINE)

1. 250 . 50
2. 362 . 01
3. ___ . __
4. ___ . __

24.	A						B	C	D		E
	DATE(S) OF SERVICE From			To			Place of Service	Type of Service	PROCEDURES, SERVICES, OR SUPPLIES (Explain Unusual Circumstances)		DIAGNOSIS CODE
	MM	DD	YY	MM	DD	YY			CPT/HCPCS	MODIFIER	
1	11	15	00				11		99213		1
2	11	15	00				11		92250		2
3											

21. DIAGNOSIS OR NATURE OF ILLNESS OR INJURY. (RELATE ITEMS 1,2,3 OR 4 TO ITEM 24E BY LINE)

1. 786 . 52
2. 413 . 9
3. 410 . 9
4. ___ . __

24.	A						B	C	D		E
	DATE(S) OF SERVICE From			To			Place of Service	Type of Service	PROCEDURES, SERVICES, OR SUPPLIES (Explain Unusual Circumstances)		DIAGNOSIS CODE
	MM	DD	YY	MM	DD	YY			CPT/HCPCS	MODIFIER	
1	11	15	00				11		71020		786.52
2	11	15	00				11		93015		413.9
3	11	15	00				11		93307		410.9

If you strongly believe that additional diagnostic information is needed by the Medicare intermediary for proper claim processing you may attach additional supporting documentation to your manual claim. Keep in mind that in most cases the additional documentation will be ignored by the claims examiners and, in other cases, will result in reimbursement delay while someone reviews your documentation.

Medicare intermediaries require that you submit claim forms using one of the above formats. Check with your local Medicare intermediary to determine which is preferred.

PENALTIES FOR NON-COMPLIANCE

The Medicare Catastrophic Coverage Act of 1988 mandates submission of an appropriate ICD-9-CM diagnosis code or codes for each procedure, service, or supply furnished by the health care professional to Medicare Part B beneficiaries. The Act further specifies that compliance is mandatory and that penalties may be assessed for noncompliance.

The penalties for noncompliance differ depending upon whether or not the health care professional has agreed to accept assignment or not.

1. Health care professionals who accept assignment on a Medicare claim and who fail to include ICD-9-CM codes as required will have their claim(s) returned for proper coding and may be subject to post-payment review by the Medicare intermediary, as well as payment denials.

2. For health care professionals who do not accept assignment, the penalties are more severe.

   A. If the original claim form does not include ICD-9-CM codes as required, and the health care professional refuses to provide the codes promptly on request to the Medicare intermediary, the professional may be subject to a civil monetary penalty in an amount not to exceed $2,000 per claim.

   B. If the health care professional continuously fails to provide ICD-9-CM codes as requested, the professional may be subject to the sanction process described in section 1842 (j) (2) (A), which mandates that the professional may be barred from participation in the Medicare program for a period not to exceed five years.

OTHER INSURANCE CLAIM ISSUES

DOWN CODING

Down coding is the process of reducing a code from one of a higher value to one of a lower value which results in lowered reimbursement. Prior to the elimination of procedure descriptions on insurance claim forms, this process resulted in the loss of millions of dollars annually by health care professionals and their patients. While down coding due to mismatch of description to code has been virtually eliminated, there are still areas where insurance carriers can find ways to reduce, delay, or deny reimbursement based upon down coding.

With diagnosis coding, the key issue is that the ICD-9-CM code(s) provide justification for the procedure, service or supply or the level of service provided. A key point to remember is that if there are any current coexisting conditions which may complicate the treatment for the primary condition, it is very important to include the ICD-9-CM codes for the coexisting conditions which will help to justify the level of service provided.

CONCURRENT CARE

Reimbursement problems often arise when a patient is being treated by different professionals within the same billing entity (medical group or clinic), for different problems at the same time. This is known as concurrent care. For example, a patient may be hospitalized by a clinic's general surgeon for an operation and may also be seen while hospitalized by the group's cardiologist for an unrelated cardiac condition.

If you submit claims for daily hospital visits by both of the above professionals without explanation, most insurance carriers would reject one daily visit as an apparent "duplication" of service. Prior to publication of the 1992 edition of CPT, the key to obtaining proper reimbursement for concurrent care was first, to use the procedure modifier -75, Concurrent Care, Services Rendered by More than One Physician, and second, to submit a different ICD-9-CM code for the services provided by each physician, which support and justify the need for those services.

Modifier -75 was deleted in the 1992 edition of CPT. Therefore, when using the new CPT Evaluation and Management codes to bill Medicare, the ICD-9-CM code becomes the key to proper reimbursement.

ELECTRONIC CLAIMS

HCFA has issued instructions to all Medicare intermediaries requiring them to make the changes necessary to accommodate the new ICD-9-CM coding requirements in the electronic billing process. ICD-9-CM codes have been required for Medicare electronic claims processing since its implementation in 1983.

Those professionals who use electronic claims processing, either with a computer billing service bureau or their own computer system, are already providing ICD-9-CM codes with their claims. However, as mentioned previously, most professionals are not coding to the degree of accuracy, certainty or specificity required by the new regulations, so review and changes to the diagnostic coding process will be required.

In addition, most previous electronic claim formats allowed diagnostic coding on a one to one basis with procedures. For example, if you listed six services or procedures in the electronic claim, you could list up to six different ICD-9-CM codes as well. Under the new format you are restricted a maximum of four ICD-9-CM codes as allowed on the HCFA1500 claim form with some provisions for listing additional diagnosis codes with the charge record as before.

In most cases, this new requirement will result in program changes by your computer billing service bureau, your computer software vendor, or in-house programming staff. In addition, you will probably need to review and revise your input documents (superbills, fee tickets, visit slips, etc.) in order to assure compliance with the new coding format.

USE OF SUPERBILLS

Health care professionals who are not participating in the Medicare program and who do not take assignment may allow Medicare beneficiaries to file their own Medicare claims. In order to expedite the claims process for unassigned Medicare beneficiaries, you must provide the patient with a Superbill (billing statement) which includes the ICD-9-CM codes listed in the proper order, along with a number next to each procedure code indicating the corresponding ICD-9-CM diagnosis code. Failure to provide this information will result in penalties as described above.

Since October 1990, health care professionals have been required to submit HCFA1500 claim forms for all Medicare patients regardless of participation status. Some have continued to attach a Superbill to the claim instead of filling out the form. As of April 1, 1992, Medicare carriers will no longer accept Superbills attached to claim forms.

ADDITIONAL INFORMATION

To avoid coding problems and to maximize reimbursement, it is important that the health care professional and his or her staff fully understand the requirements of the Medicare regulations and the fundamentals of the ICD-9-CM coding system. Health care professionals may need to become more personally involved in the area of diagnostic coding as well as reviewing the accuracy and precision of the diagnostic statements in their medical records.

In addition to publications such as this one, many local, regional and national firms provide self-study books and tapes, seminars, and consulting services to help you learn more about ICD-9-CM coding. Contact your local, state or national medical association and/or your local Medicare intermediary for additional information regarding these services.

UNDERSTANDING ICD-9-CM

ICD-9-CM is an acronym for *International Classification of Diseases, 9th Revision, Clinical Modification*, published under different names since 1900. ICD-9-CM is a statistical classification system which arranges diseases and injuries into groups according to established criteria. Most ICD-9-CM codes are numeric and consist of three, four or five numbers and a description. The codes are revised approximately every 10 years by the World Health Organization and annual updates are published by HCFA.

HISTORICAL PERSPECTIVE

The *International Classification of Diseases, 9th Revision, Clinical Modification* (ICD-9-CM) is based on the official version of the World Health Organization's (WHO) 9th Revision, International Classification of Diseases (ICD-9). ICD-9 is designed for the classification of morbidity and mortality information for statistical purposes, for the indexing of medical records by disease and operations, and for data storage and retrieval. ICD-9-CM replaced the Eighth Revision International Classification of Diseases, Adapted for Use in the United States, commonly referred to as ICDA.

The concept of extending the International Classification of Diseases for use in hospital indexing was originally developed in response to a need for a more efficient basis for storage and retrieval of diagnostic data. In 1950, the U.S. Public Health Service and the Veterans Administration began independent tests of the International Classification of Diseases for hospital indexing purposes. In the following year, the Columbia Presbyterian Medical Center in New York City adopted the International Classification of Diseases, 6th Revision for use in its medical record department. A few years later, the Commission on Professional and Hospital Activities adopted the International Classification of Diseases for use in hospitals participating in the Professional Activity Study (PAS).

In view of the growing interest in the use of the International Classification of Diseases for hospital indexing, a study was undertaken in 1956 by the American Medical Association and the American Medical Record Association of the relative efficiencies of coding systems for diagnostic indexing. Following this study, the major uses of the International Classification of Diseases for hospital indexing purposes consolidated their experiences and an adaptation was published in December 1959. A revision containing the first "Classification of Operations and Treatments" was published in 1962.

In 1968, following a study by the American Hospital Association, the United States Public Health Service published the Eighth Revision International Classification of Diseases, Adapted for Use in the United States. This publication became commonly known as ICDA, and served as the basis for coding diagnostic data for official morbidity and mortality statistics in the United States.

ICD-9-CM BACKGROUND

In February 1977, a committee was convened by the National Center for Health Statistics to provide advice and counsel for the development of clinical modification of the ICD-9. The organizations represented on the committee included:

- American Association of Health Data Systems
- American Hospital Association
- American Medical Record Association
- Association for Health Records
- Council on Clinical Classifications, sponsored by:
    - American Academy of Pediatrics
    - American College of Obstetricians and Gynecologists
    - American College of Physicians
    - American College of Surgeons
    - American Psychiatric Association
- Commission on Professional and Hospital Activities
- Health Care Financing Administration
- WHO Center for Classification of Diseases

The resulting ICD-9-CM is a clinical modification of the World Health Organization's International Classification of Diseases, 9th Revision (ICD-9). The term "clinical" is used to emphasize the modifications intent; namely, to serve as a useful tool in the area of classification of morbidity data for indexing of medical records, medical care review, ambulatory and other medical care programs, as well as for basic health statistics.

In use since January 1979, ICD-9-CM provides a diagnostic coding system which is more precise than those needed only for statistical groupings and trend analysis. Official addenda (updates) to ICD-9-CM were issued in October 1986, 1987 and 1988 by the Health Care Financing Administration. A special addendum was published by the U.S. Public Health Service in January 1988 containing codes for AIDS and AIDS related illnesses.

USE OF ICD-9-CM CODES FOR PROFESSIONAL BILLING

Until passage of the Medicare Catastrophic Coverage Act of 1988, health care professionals were not required to report ICD-9-CM codes when billing government or private insurance carriers for reimbursement. The exception to this requirement was for those health care professionals who filed insurance claims electronically and those who used "code driven" computer billing services or computer systems.

Most health care professionals simply included the text or description of the injury, illness, sign or symptom which was the reason for the encounter. Insurance carriers who used ICD-9-CM coding had to code the diagnostic statements prior to input into their computer systems for reimbursement processing.

A specific requirement of the Medicare Catastrophic Coverage Act of 1988 required health care professionals to include ICD-9-CM codes on their Medicare claim forms effective April 1, 1989. A two-month grace period, to June 1, 1989, was implemented at the request of the American Medical Association, to allow health care professionals additional time to develop the knowledge and systems necessary to implement the requirement.

In the area of issues related to reimbursement, rules and regulations mandated by HCFA for the Medicare program traditionally are soon followed by similar rules for the Medicaid program and private insurance carriers.

ICD-10

The World Health Organization (WHO) traditionally releases a new revision of ICD about every 10 years. ICD-10 was originally expected in 1990 or 1991; however, it was not released by the WHO until 1992. ICD-10 was published as a three-volume set that includes the diagnostic codes with descriptions, an instructional text, and an alphabetic index.

To increase the utility of ICD for reporting morbidity and mortality statistics and to increase the number of codes, WHO made major changes to ICD-10. The most significant change is that all numeric diagnosis codes in ICD-9 were changed to alphanumeric codes in ICD-10. All diagnosis codes in ICD-10 have a letter prefix.

IMPLEMENTATION SCHEDULE

After WHO releases a new edition of ICD, the work undergoes an extensive review and revision in the United States by the healthcare industry. Representatives from HCFA, the Department of Health and Human Services, the insurance industry, physician's associations and hospital associations review and revise ICD and eventually publish as the "Clinical Modification" of the current edition of ICD. This revision includes the modification of terminology from British English to United States English, and other revisions designed to incorporate current medical technology and health insurance industry practices in the United States.

Following release of ICD-10 in 1992, the original plan was that ICD-CM would be released in the United States by the year 2000. However, the review process took longer than expected and the release date was changed to 2001. In addition, the committee responsible for making these modifications recommended an increase in the number of digits in the diagnosis coding system, which would allow more codes to be defined. However, this modification would also require the reprogramming of every computer system in the United States that processes diagnosis codes, at a potential cost of millions or billions of dollars for physicians, hospitals, and government agencies.

In October 1999, HCFA announced that due to the administrative simplification requirements of Section 262 of the Health Insurance Portability and Accountability Act of 1996 (Public Law 104-191), implementation of ICD-10-CM was indefinitely delayed and the current thinking was no longer "when" the new code system would be implemented, but "if" the new code system would be implemented. As a result of this decision, ICD-9-CM will continue to be the diagnostic coding system of choice for the next few years.

TERMINOLOGY

There are terms used throughout this publication that are important for a proper understanding of ICD-9-CM. The following terms are defined specifically as they are used for ICD-9-CM with the knowledge that some terms may have other definitions and meanings.

Acute refers to the condition which is the primary reason for the current encounter.

Addenda official updates to ICD-9-CM published in October of each year since 1986.

Adverse any response to a drug which is noxious and unintended and occurs with proper dosage.

Aftercare an encounter for something planned in advance, for example, cast removal.

AHFS American Hospital Formulary Service.

Alphabetic the portion of ICD-9-CM which lists definitions and codes in alphabetic order. Also referred to as Volume 2.

Category refers to diagnoses codes listed within a specific three-digit category, for example category 250, Diabetes Mellitus.

Cause that which brings about any condition or produces any effect.

Chronic continuing over a long period of time or recurring frequently.

Coding the process of transferring written or verbal descriptions of diseases, injuries and procedures into numerical designations.

Combination a code which combines a diagnosis with an associated secondary process or complication.

Complication the occurrence of two or more diseases in the same patient at the same time.

Concurrent Care when a patient is being treated by more than one provider for different conditions at the same time.

Conventions refers to the use of certain abbreviations, punctuation, symbols, type faces, and other instructions which must be clearly understood in order to use ICD-9-CM.

CPT Current Procedural Terminology. Listing of codes and descriptions for procedures, services and supplies published by the American Medical Association. Used to bill insurance carriers.

Diagnosis a written description of the reason(s) for the procedure, service, supply or encounter.

Diagnostic Statement see DIAGNOSIS

Down Coding the process where insurance carriers reduce the value of a procedure, and the resulting reimbursement.

E Codes specific ICD-9-CM codes used to identify the cause of injury, poisoning and other adverse effects.

Eponyms medical procedures or conditions named after a person or a place.

Etiology the cause(s) or origin of a disease.

Fee Ticket See SUPERBILL.

HCFA Health Care Financing Administration. The government agency which administers the Medicare and Medicaid programs.

HCFA1500 Uniform Health Insurance Claim Form used for billing services to Medicare and other insurance carriers.

Hierarchy a system which ranks items one above another.

ICD-9-CM International Classification of Diseases, 9th Revision, Clinical Modification.

ICD-10 International Classification of Diseases, 10th Revision

Late Effect a residual effect (condition produced) after the acute phase of an illness or injury has ended.

Main Term refers to listings in the Alphabetic Index appearing BOLDFACE type.

Manifestation characteristic signs or symptoms of an illness.

Multiple Coding refers to the need to use more than one ICD-9-CM code to fully identify a condition.

Primary Code the ICD-9-CM code which defines the main reason for the current encounter.

Residual the long-term condition(s) resulting from a previous acute illness or injury.

Rule Out refers to a method used to indicate that a condition is probable, suspected, or questionable but unconfirmed. ICD-9-CM has no provisions for the use of this term.

Secondary Code code(s) listed after the primary code which further indicate the cause(s) for the current encounter or define the need for higher levels of care.

Sections refers to portions of the Tabular List which are organized in groups of three-digit code numbers. For example, Malignant Neoplasm of Lip, Oral Cavity and Pharynx (140-149).

Sequencing the process of listing ICD-9-CM codes in the proper order.

Specificity refers to the requirement to code to the highest number of digits possible, 3, 4 or 5, when choosing an ICD-9-CM code.

Sub Term refers to listings appearing in the Alphabetic Index under MAIN TERMS and always indented two spaces to the right.

Subcategories refers to groupings of four-digit codes listed under three-digit categories.

Superbill an encounter form designed to record procedures, services and supplies along with corresponding diagnostic information.

Tabular List the portion of ICD-9-CM which lists codes and definitions in numeric order. Also referred to as Volume 1.

V Codes specific ICD-9-CM codes used to identify encounters for reasons other than illness or injury, for example, immunization.

Volume 1 see TABULAR LIST

Volume 2 see ALPHABETIC INDEX

Volume 3 procedure codes used only for hospital coding. Volume 3 contains both a numeric listing and alphabetic index. These codes are now maintained by the American Health Information Management Association (AHIMA).

IMPORTANT CODING AND BILLING ISSUES

DIAGNOSIS CODES MUST SUPPORT PROCEDURE CODES

Each service or procedure performed for a patient should be represented by a diagnosis that would substantiate those particular services or procedures as necessary in the investigation or treatment of their condition based on currently accepted standards of practice by the medical profession.

EXAMPLE: A patient comes into the office complaining of difficulty breathing, congestion, and fever. After the physician examines the patient, physical findings suggest the possibility of pneumonia. In the meantime, the patient also complains of knee soreness. The physician orders the following: chest x-ray, antibiotic therapy, knee x-ray. The physician lists the diagnosis on the patient's file/superbill as Pneumonia. The biller sends out the bill with the appropriate CPT codes for office visit, chest x-ray, knee x-ray with the diagnosis of Pneumonia.

PROBLEM: The insurance claims examiner will not be able to associate the need for the knee x-ray with the diagnosis that has been reported, and therefore denies that particular service.

SOLUTION: The biller should have requested some type of diagnosis to substantiate the knee x-ray. What did the physician suspect or want to rule out? This then could have been coded and listed on the initial claim to prevent the claim from being held up or partially denied.

PLACE (LOCATION) OF SERVICE

The actual setting that the services are rendered in for particular diagnoses plays an important part in reimbursement. Many people became accustomed to using Emergency Rooms for any type of illness or injury. By utilizing highly specialized places of service for conditions that were not true emergencies, third party payer were being billed with CPT codes indicating emergency services were rendered. Since the cost of services rendered on an emergency basis is considerably more expensive than those services in an non-emergency situation, third party payers began watching for those claims with diagnoses that did not indicate that a true emergency existed. Payment then was based on what the cost would have been had the patient been treated in the proper setting.

EXAMPLE: A patient comes to an emergency room for treatment of a sore throat and cough. The physician examines the patient and recommends several prescriptions.
The diagnosis recorded is that of Upper Respiratory Infection.

PROBLEM: The claim is prepared and submitted to the third party payer for consideration with the CPT code indicating E.R. visit and the diagnosis of U.R.I. The payment is reduced to what it would have cost if the services had been rendered in the office place of service.

SOLUTION: Educate your patients that emergency rooms should only be utilized for true emergency situations. Let them know that their insurance may pay less for a non-emergency situation treated in an emergency room setting and that they may be responsible for any balance not paid by their insurance carrier. Some practices have also extended their office hours to include Saturdays and evenings to help alleviate this problem.

LEVEL OF SERVICE PROVIDED

The patient's condition and the treatment of that condition must be billed according to the criteria, as published by the AMA, for each level of service (i.e., minimal, brief, limited, intermediate, extended, comprehensive). Many practices bill the office visit level that they know will pay better rather than to consider the criteria that must be met to use a particular level of service. Again, the patient's diagnosis enters into this concept as well, since it is often the diagnosis that indicates the complexity of the level of service to be used.

EXAMPLE: A patient comes into the office with the symptoms of an Acute Respiratory Infection. The physician reviews past medical management of previous U.R.I.'s to determine the effectiveness of that treatment. He prescribes what medication he feels should be effective for the patient's condition. The claim is then submitted indicating an intermediate level of service.

PROBLEM: Since the criteria for an intermediate level of service include the evaluation of a new or existing condition complicated with a new diagnostic or management problem, it is possible for the third party payer to reduce the payment to the limited level of service someone with the reported condition of U.R.I.

SOLUTION: Become aware of what criteria must be met in order to bill for a certain level of service. Again, this means an education process, but this time, for the provider rather than the patient.

FREQUENCY OF SERVICES

Many times claims are submitted for a patient with the same diagnosis and the same procedure(s) time after time. When the diagnosis indicates a chronic condition and the claims do not indicate any change in the patient's treatment or give any indication that the patient's condition has been altered (i.e., exacerbated, other symptomology), the third party payer may deny payment based on the frequency of services for the reported condition.

EXAMPLE: A longstanding patient comes in for an office visit. This patient has a history of COPD and comes in the office every 2-3 weeks. Every claim that you submit for consideration had the ICD-9-CM code indicating COPD. Also, there never seems to be any other service rendered.

PROBLEM: The third party payer notices the repeated service for the same chronic condition. Based on the information for the present claim and previous claims, the payer may request further information or deny payment.

SOLUTION: Check with the physician from time to time to see if, in fact, the patient may have come in for another reason. <u>Do not copy the information from the previous claim(s) automatically</u>. Verify the diagnostic information for each visit. NOTE: this patient may have come in with Acute Bronchitis. The physician may have only charged for the office visit and given the patient prescriptions. In this case, the claim should be coded for Acute Bronchitis (primary diagnosis) and COPD (secondary diagnosis). This would eliminate any chance of denial based on frequency for the reported condition.

Currently, statistics are being tabulated from all claims submitted to Medicare or any other third party payer. These statistics will be used in the future as the basis of your fee profile for a prospective payment system. Again, this is why correct reporting by using the most appropriate codes is very important to the financial outlook of a provider.

FORMAT OF ICD-9-CM

The *International Classification of Diseases, 9th Revision, Clinical Modification* was originally published as a three volume set (2nd edition). Newer versions of ICD-9-CM, Fifth Edition, are available as two separate books (Volume 1 and Volume 2) and as a single book containing Volume 1 and Volume 2, or Volumes 1, 2 and 3 depending on the publisher.

The Third Edition of ICD-9-CM includes all official addenda from October 1986 through October 1988. The Fourth Edition of ICD-9-CM includes all official addenda from October 1986 through October 1991. Most publishers who print the ICD-9-CM now offer an annual version, usually published in December of each year, which includes all of the addenda through October of the same year.

THE TABULAR LIST (VOLUME 1)

The Tabular List (Volume 1) is a numeric listing of diagnosis codes and descriptions consisting of 17 chapters which classify diseases and injuries, two sections containing supplementary codes (V codes and E codes) and six appendices.

CLASSIFICATION OF DISEASES AND INJURIES

The Classification of Diseases and Injuries includes the following 17 chapters:

Chapter 1 Infectious and Parasitic Diseases (001-139)

Chapter 2 Neoplasms (140-239)

Chapter 3 Endocrine, Nutritional and Metabolic Diseases, and Immunity Disorders (240-279)

Chapter 4 Diseases of the Blood and Blood-Forming Organs (280-289)

Chapter 5 Mental Disorders (290-319)

Chapter 6 Diseases of the Nervous System and Sense Organs (320-389)

Chapter 7 Diseases of the Circulatory System (390-459)

Chapter 8 Diseases of the Respiratory System (460-519)

Chapter 9 Diseases of the Digestive System (520-579)

Chapter 10 Diseases of the Genitourinary System (580-629)

Chapter 11 Complications of Pregnancy, Childbirth, and the Puerperium (630-677)

Chapter 12 Diseases of the Skin and Subcutaneous Tissue (680-709)

Chapter 13 Diseases of the Musculoskeletal System and Connective Tissue (710-739)

Chapter 14 Congenital Anomalies (740-759)

Chapter 15 Certain Conditions Originating in the Perinatal Period (760-779)

Chapter 16 Symptoms, Signs and Ill-defined Conditions (780-799)

Chapter 17 Injury and Poisoning (800-999)

Each chapter of the Tabular List (Volume 1) is structured into four components; namely:

Sections: groups of three-digit code numbers

Categories: three-digit code numbers

Subcategories: four-digit code numbers

Fifth-Digit Subclassifications: five-digit code numbers

SUPPLEMENTARY CLASSIFICATIONS

There are two supplementary classifications included in the Tabular List (Volume 1). These are:

V Codes — Supplementary Classification of Factors Influencing Health Status and Contact with Health Services (V01-V82)

E Codes — Supplementary Classification of External Causes of Injury and Poisoning (E800-E999)

APPENDICES

The Tabular List (Volume 1) includes five appendices. These are:

Appendix 1 — Morphology of Neoplasms

Appendix 2 — Glossary of Mental Disorders

Appendix 3 — Classification of Drugs by American Hospital Formulary Service List Number and their ICD-9-CM Equivalents

Appendix 4 — Classification of Industrial Accidents According to Agency

Appendix 5 — List of Three-Digit Categories

THE ALPHABETICAL INDEX (VOLUME 2)

The Alphabetic Index (Volume 2) of ICD-9-CM consists of an alphabetic list of terms and codes, two supplementary sections following the alphabetic listing, plus two special tables found within the alphabetic listing. The Alphabetic Index (Volume 2) is structured as follows:

MAIN TERMS: — appear in **BOLDFACE** type

SUBTERMS: — are always indented two spaces to the right under main terms

CARRY-OVER LINES: are always indented more than two spaces from the level of the preceding line

SUPPLEMENTARY SECTIONS

The supplementary sections following the Alphabetic Index are:

TABLE OF DRUGS AND CHEMICALS

This table contains a classification of drugs and other chemical substances to identify poisoning states and external causes of adverse effects.

INDEX TO EXTERNAL CAUSES OF INJURIES & POISONINGS (E-CODES)

This section contains the index to the codes which classify environmental events, circumstances, and other conditions as the cause of injury and other adverse effects.

SPECIAL TABLES

The two special tables, located within the Alphabetic Index, and found under the main terms as underlined below, are the:

Hypertension Table
Neoplasm Table

PROCEDURES: TABULAR LIST AND ALPHABETIC INDEX (VOLUME 3)

The Procedures: Tabular List and Alphabetic Index (Volume 3) consists of two sections of codes which define procedures instead of diagnoses. Frequently used incorrectly by health care professionals, codes from Volume 3 are intended only for use by hospitals. The fourth and subsequent editions of ICD-9-CM printed by the U.S. Government Printing Office did not include Volume 3.

TABULAR LIST OF PROCEDURES

Includes 16 chapters containing codes and descriptions for surgical procedures and miscellaneous diagnostic and therapeutic procedures.

ALPHABETIC INDEX TO PROCEDURES

Provides an alphabetic index to the Tabular List of Volume 3

CONVENTIONS

The ICD-9-CM Tabular List (Volume 1) makes use of certain abbreviations, punctuation, symbols, and other conventions which must be clearly understood. The purpose of these conventions is first, to provide special coding instructions, and second, to conserve space.

INSTRUCTIONAL TERMS

Instructional terms define what is, or what is not, included in a given subdivision. This is accomplished by using both inclusion and exclusion terms.

INCLUDES: Indicates separate terms as modifying adjectives, sites and conditions, entered under a subdivision, such as a category, to further define or give examples of the content of the category.

Excludes Exclusion terms are enclosed in a box and are printed in italics to draw attention to their presence. The importance of this instructional term is its use as a guideline to direct the coder to the proper code assignment. In other words, all terms following the word EXCLUDES: are to be coded elsewhere as indicated in each instance.

NOTES These are used to define terms and give coding instructions. Often used to list the fifth-digit subclassifications for certain categories.

SEE	Acts as a cross reference and is an explicit direction to look elsewhere. This instructional term must *always* be followed. (Cross references provide the user with other possible modifiers for a term, or its synonyms.)
SEE CATEGORY	A variation of the instructional term SEE. This refers the coder to a specific category. You must *always* follow this instructional term.
SEE ALSO	A direction given to look elsewhere if the main term or subterm(s) are not sufficient to code the information you have.
CODE FIRST	Identifies those codes not intended to be used as a principal diagnosis or not to be sequenced before the underlying diseases.
USE ADDITIONAL CODE	Adds information which results in a better understanding of the diagnosis.

PUNCTUATION MARKS

( )	PARENTHESIS are used to enclose supplementary words which may be present or absent in a statement of disease without effecting the code assignment.
[ ]	SQUARE BRACKETS are used to enclose synonyms, alternate wordings or explanatory phrases.
:	COLONS are used after an incomplete phrase or term which requires one or more of the modifiers indented under it to make it assignable to a given category. EXCEPTION to this rule pertains to the abbreviation NOS.

{ } — BRACES are used to connect a series of terms to a common stem. Each term on the left of the brace is incomplete and must be completed by a term to the right of the brace.

ABBREVIATIONS

NOS — Not Otherwise Specified. Equivalent to Unspecified. This abbreviation refers to a lack of sufficient detail in the statement of diagnosis to be able to assign it to a more specific sub division within the classification.

NEC — Not Elsewhere Classified. Used with ill-defined terms to alert the coder that a specified form of the condition is classified differently. The category number for the term including NEC is to be used only when the coder lacks the information necessary to code the term to a more specific category.

SYMBOLS

□ — The LOZENGE symbol appearing in the left margin preceding a four-digit code indicates that the code and description are not the same in ICD-9-CM as in ICD-9. May be ignored for coding purposes.

RELATED TERMS

AND — Whenever this term appears in a title, it should be interpreted as "and/or."

WITH — When this term is used in a title it indicates a requirement that both parts of the title must be present in the diagnostic statement.

ANATOMICAL ILLUSTRATIONS

A fundamental knowledge and understanding of basic human anatomy and physiology is a prerequisite for accurate diagnosis coding. While a comprehensive treatment of anatomy and physiology is beyond the scope of this text, the large scale, full color anatomical illustrations on the following pages are designed to facilitate the diagnosis coding process for both beginning and experienced coders.

The illustrations provide an anatomical perspective of diagnosis coding by providing a side-by-side view of the major systems of the human body and a corresponding list of the most common diagnoses categories used to support medical, surgical and diagnostic services performed on the illustrated system.

The diagnostic categories listed on the left facing page of each anatomical illustration are three-digit categories and may not be used for coding. These categories are provided as "pointers" to the appropriate section of the ICD-9-CM Volume 1 where the complete listings, including 4th and 5th digits if appropriate, may be found.

ICD-9-CM ANATOMICAL ILLUSTRATIONS

PLATE 1. SKIN AND SUBCUTANEOUS TISSUE-MALE

Viral diseases accompanied by exanthem	050-057
Neoplasms	
Malignant melanoma of skin	172
Other malignant neoplasm of skin	173
Malignant neoplasm of male breast	175
Kaposi's sarcoma	176
Benign neoplasm of skin	216
Carcinoma in situ of skin	232
Infections of skin and subcutaneous tissue	
Carbuncle and furuncle	680
Cellulitis and abscess of finger and toe	681
Other cellulitis and abscess	682
Acute lymphadenitis	683
Impetigo	684
Pilonidal cyst	685
Other local infections of skin and subcutaneous tissue	686
Other inflammatory conditions of skin and subcutaneous tissue	
Erythematosquamous dermatosis	690
Atopic dermatitis and related conditions	691
Contact dermatitis and other eczema	692
Dermatitis due to substances taken internally	693
Bullous dermatoses	694
Erythematous conditions	695
Psoriasis and similar disorders	696
Lichen	697
Pruritus and related conditions	698
Other diseases of skin and subcutaneous tissue	
Corns and callosities	700
Other hypertrophic and atrophic conditions of skin	701
Diseases of nail	703
Diseases of hair and hair follicles	704
Disorders of sweat glands	705
Diseases of sebaceous glands	706
Chronic ulcer of skin	707
Urticaria	708
Other disorders of skin and subcutaneous tissue	709
Symptoms involving skin and other integumentary tissue	782
Symptoms, signs and ill-defined conditions	780-799

Male Figure
(Anterior View)

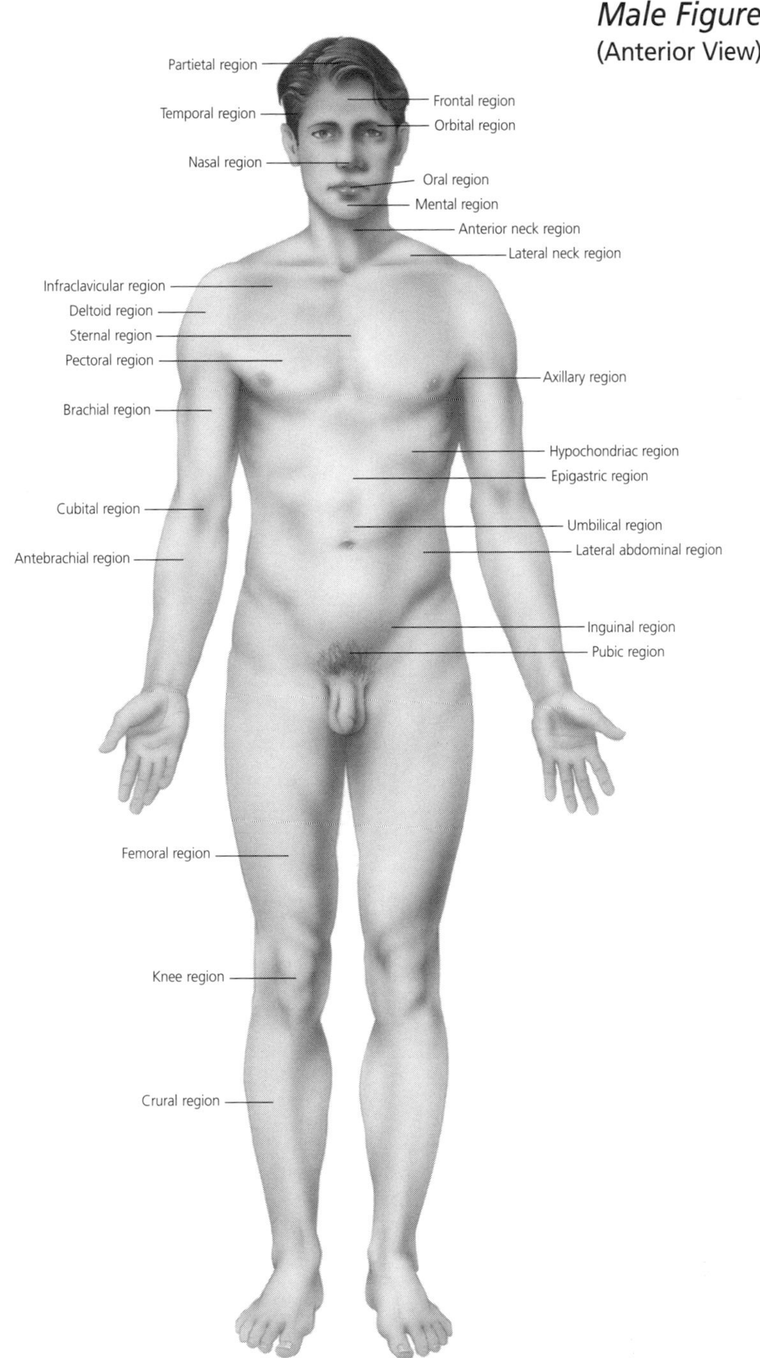

©Practice Management Information Corp., Los Angeles, CA

PLATE 2. SKIN AND SUBCUTANEOUS TISSUE - FEMALE

Viral diseases accompanied by exanthem	050-057
Neoplasms	
Malignant melanoma of skin	172
Other malignant neoplasm of skin	173
Malignant neoplasm of female breast	174
Kaposi's sarcoma	176
Benign neoplasm of skin	216
Carcinoma in situ of skin	232
Infections of skin and subcutaneous tissue	
Carbuncle and furuncle	680
Cellulitis and abscess of finger and toe	681
Other cellulitis and abscess	682
Acute lymphadenitis	683
Impetigo	684
Pilonidal cyst	685
Other local infections of skin and subcutaneous tissue	686
Other inflammatory conditions of skin and subcutaneous tissue	
Erythematosquamous dermatosis	690
Atopic dermatitis and related conditions	691
Contact dermatitis and other eczema	692
Dermatitis due to substances taken internally	693
Bullous dermatoses	694
Erythematous conditions	695
Psoriasis and similar disorders	696
Lichen	697
Pruritus and related conditions	698
Other diseases of skin and subcutaneous tissue	
Corns and callosities	700
Other hypertrophic and atrophic conditions of skin	701
Other dermatoses	702
Diseases of nail	703
Diseases of hair and hair follicles	704
Disorders of sweat glands	705
Diseases of sebaceous glands	706
Chronic ulcer of skin	707
Urticaria	708
Other disorders of skin and subcutaneous tissue	709
Symptoms involving skin and other integumentary tissue	782
Symptoms, signs and ill-defined conditions	780-799

Female Figure
(Anterior View)

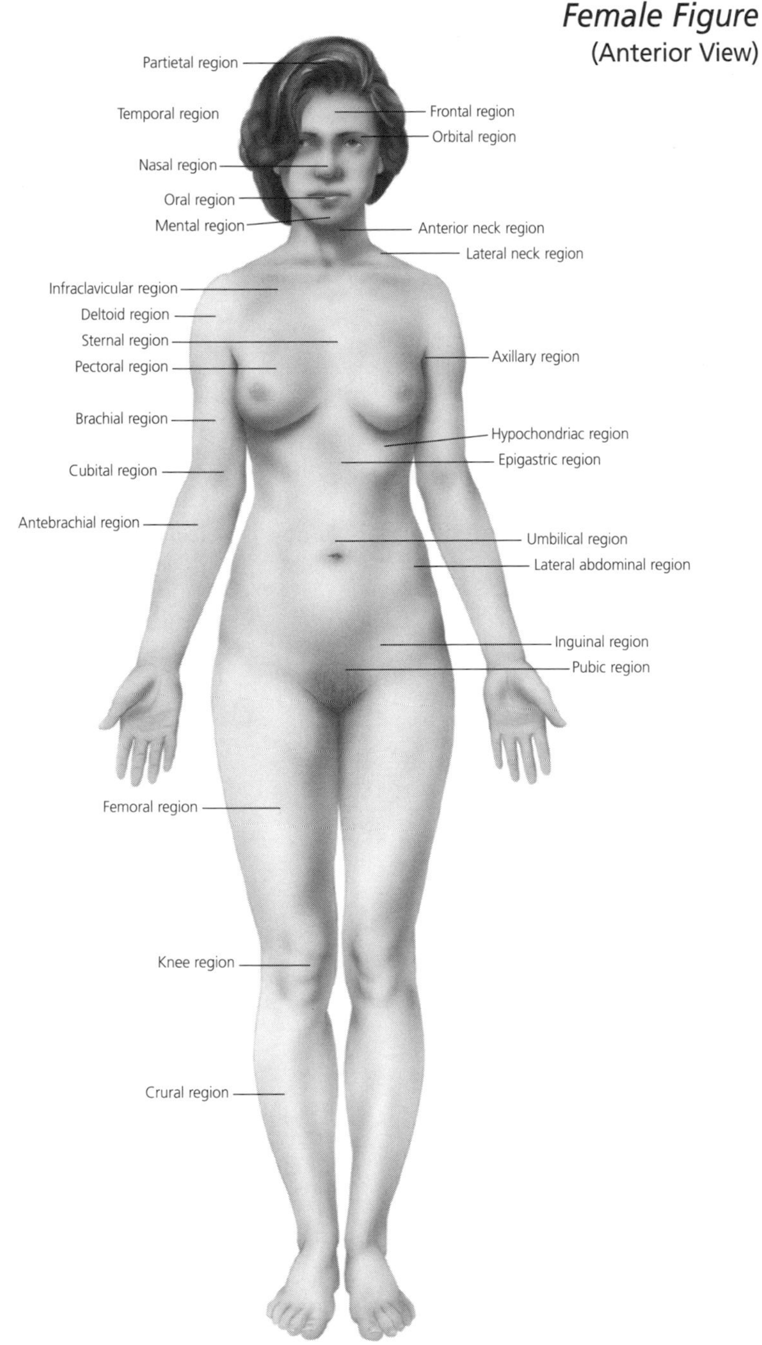

©Practice Management Information Corp., Los Angeles, CA

PLATE 3. FEMALE BREAST

Malignant neoplasm of bone, connective tissue, skin, and breast

Malignant neoplasm of female breast	174
Benign neoplasm of breast	217
Carcinoma in situ of breast and genitourinary system	233

Disorders of breast

Benign mammary dysplasias	610
Other disorders of breast	611

Complications of the puerperium

Infections of the breast and nipple associated with childbirth	675
Other disorders of the breast associated with childbirth, and disorders of lactation	676

Symptoms, signs and ill-defined conditions 780-799

Persons without reported diagnosis encountered during examination

Observation and evaluation for suspected conditions not found	V71
Special screening for malignant neoplasms	V76

Female Breast

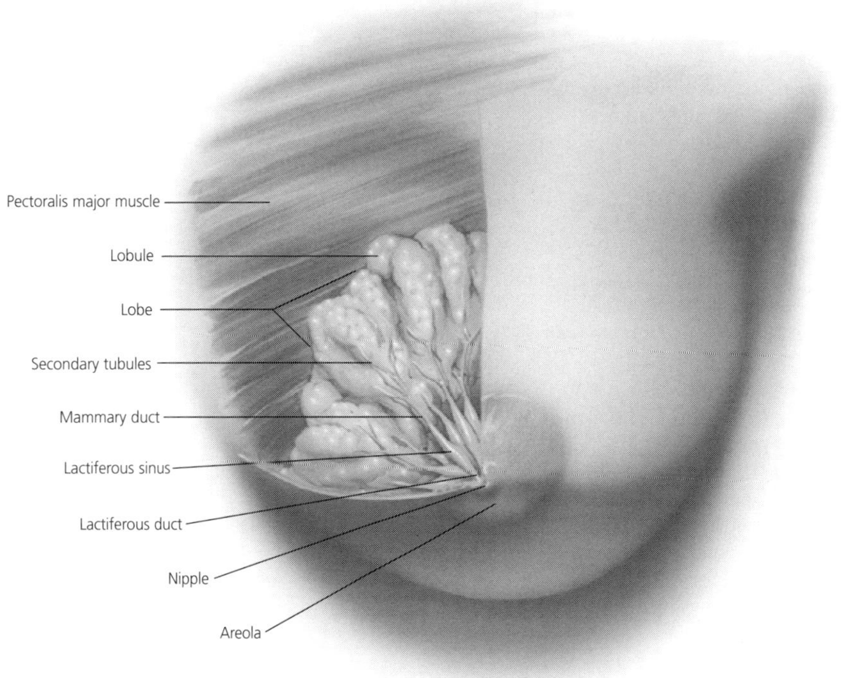

©Practice Management Information Corp., Los Angeles, CA

PLATE 4. MUSCULAR SYSTEM AND CONNECTIVE TISSUE - ANTERIOR VIEW

Arthropathies and related disorders

Diffuse diseases of connective tissue	710
Arthropathy associated with infections	711
Crystal arthropathies	712
Arthropathy associated with other disorders classified elsewhere	713
Rheumatoid arthritis and other inflammatory polyarthropathies	714
Osteoarthrosis and allied disorders	715
Internal derangement of knee	717
Other derangement of joint	718

Dorsopathies

Ankylosing spondylitis and other inflammatory spondylopathies	720
Spondylosis and allied disorders	721
Intervertebral disc disorders	722
Other disorders of cervical region	723

Rheumatism, excluding the back

Polymyalgia rheumatica	725
Peripheral enthesopathies and allied syndromes	726
Other disorders of synovium, tendon, and bursa	727
Disorders of muscle, ligament, and fascia	728
Other disorders of soft tissues	729

Osteopathies, chondropathies, and acquired musculoskeletal deformities

Osteomyelitis, periostitis, and other infections involving bone	730
Osteitis deformans and osteopathies associated with other disorders classified elsewhere	731
Osteochondropathies	732
Flat foot	734
Acquired deformities of toe	735
Other acquired deformities of limbs	736
Curvature of spine	737
Other acquired deformity	738
Nonallopathic lesions, not elsewhere classified	739

Symptoms, signs and ill-defined conditions 780-799

Muscular System
(Anterior View)

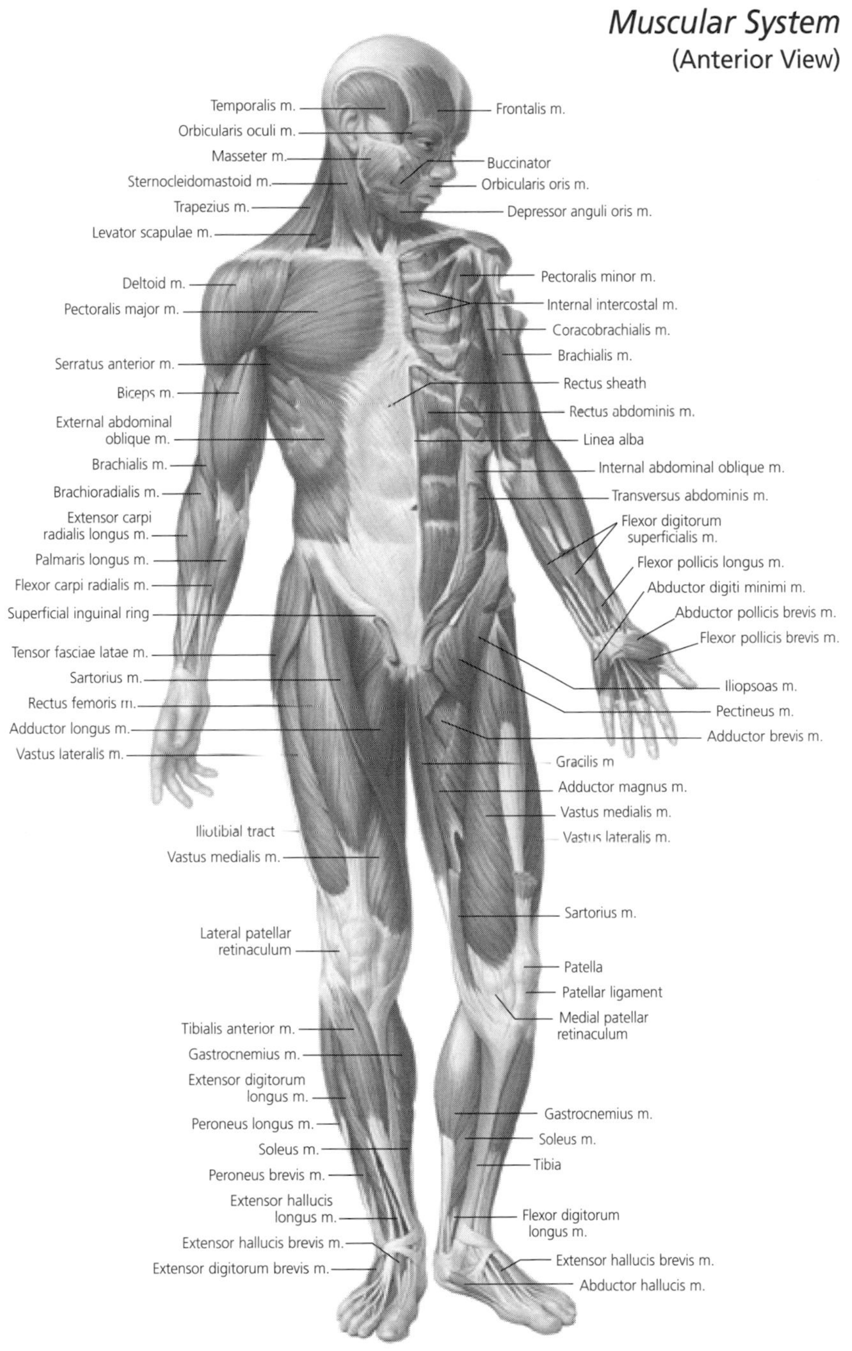

©Scientific Publishing Ltd., Rolling Meadows, IL

PLATE 5. MUSCULAR SYSTEM AND CONNECTIVE TISSUE - POSTERIOR VIEW

Arthropathies and related disorders

Diffuse diseases of connective tissue	710
Arthropathy associated with infections	711
Crystal arthropathies	712
Arthropathy associated with other disorders classified elsewhere	713
Rheumatoid arthritis and other inflammatory polyarthropathies	714
Osteoarthrosis and allied disorders	715
Other and unspecified arthropathies	716
Internal derangement of knee	717
Other derangement of joint	718
Other and unspecified disorder of joint	719

Dorsopathies

Ankylosing spondylitis and other inflammatory spondylopathies	720
Spondylosis and allied disorders	721
Intervertebral disc disorders	722
Other disorders of cervical region	723
Other and unspecified disorders of back	724

Rheumatism, excluding the back

Polymyalgia rheumatica	725
Peripheral enthesopathies and allied syndromes	726
Other disorders of synovium, tendon, and bursa	727
Disorders of muscle, ligament, and fascia	728
Other disorders of soft tissues	729

Osteopathies, chondropathies, and acquired musculoskeletal deformities

Osteomyelitis, periostitis, and other infections involving bone	730
Osteitis deformans and osteopathies associated with other disorders classified elsewhere	731
Osteochondropathies	732
Other disorders of bone and cartilage	733
Flat foot	734
Acquired deformities of toe	735
Other acquired deformities of limbs	736
Curvature of spine	737
Other acquired deformity	738
Nonallopathic lesions, not elsewhere classified	739

Symptoms, signs and ill-defined conditions 780-799

Muscular System
(Posterior View)

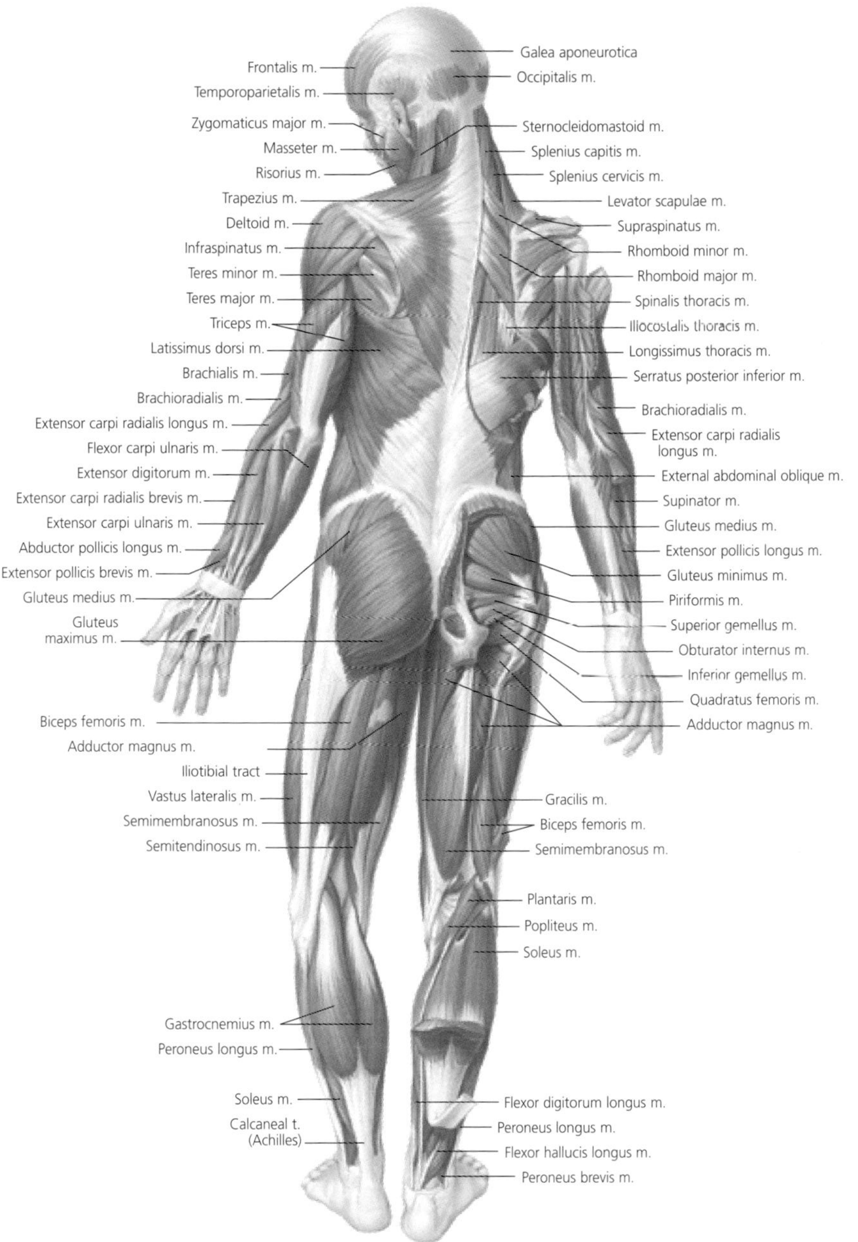

©Practice Management Information Corp., Los Angeles, CA

PLATE 6. MUSCULAR SYSTEM - SHOULDER AND ELBOW

Arthropathies and related disorders

Diffuse diseases of connective tissue	710
Arthropathy associated with infections	711
Crystal arthropathies	712
Arthropathy associated with other disorders classified elsewhere	713
Rheumatoid arthritis and other inflammatory polyarthropathies	714
Osteoarthrosis and allied disorders	715
Other and unspecified arthropathies	716
Internal derangement of knee	717
Other derangement of joint	718
Other and unspecified disorder of joint	719

Dorsopathies

Ankylosing spondylitis and other inflammatory spondylopathies	720
Spondylosis and allied disorders	721
Intervertebral disc disorders	722
Other disorders of cervical region	723
Other and unspecified disorders of back	724

Rheumatism, excluding the back

Polymyalgia rheumatica	725
Peripheral enthesopathies and allied syndromes	726
Other disorders of synovium, tendon, and bursa	727
Disorders of muscle, ligament, and fascia	728
Other disorders of soft tissues	729

Osteopathies, chondropathies, and acquired musculoskeletal deformities

Osteomyelitis, periostitis, and other infections involving bone	730
Osteitis deformans and osteopathies associated with other disorders classified elsewhere	731
Osteochondropathies	732
Other disorders of bone and cartilage	733
Flat foot	734
Acquired deformities of toe	735
Other acquired deformities of limbs	736
Curvature of spine	737
Other acquired deformity	738
Nonallopathic lesions, not elsewhere classified	739

Symptoms, signs and ill-defined conditions 780-799

Sprains and strains of joints and adjacent muscles

Sprains and strains of shoulder and upper arm	840
Sprains and strains of elbow and forearm	841
Other and ill-defined sprains and strains	848

Shoulder and Elbow

(Anterior View)

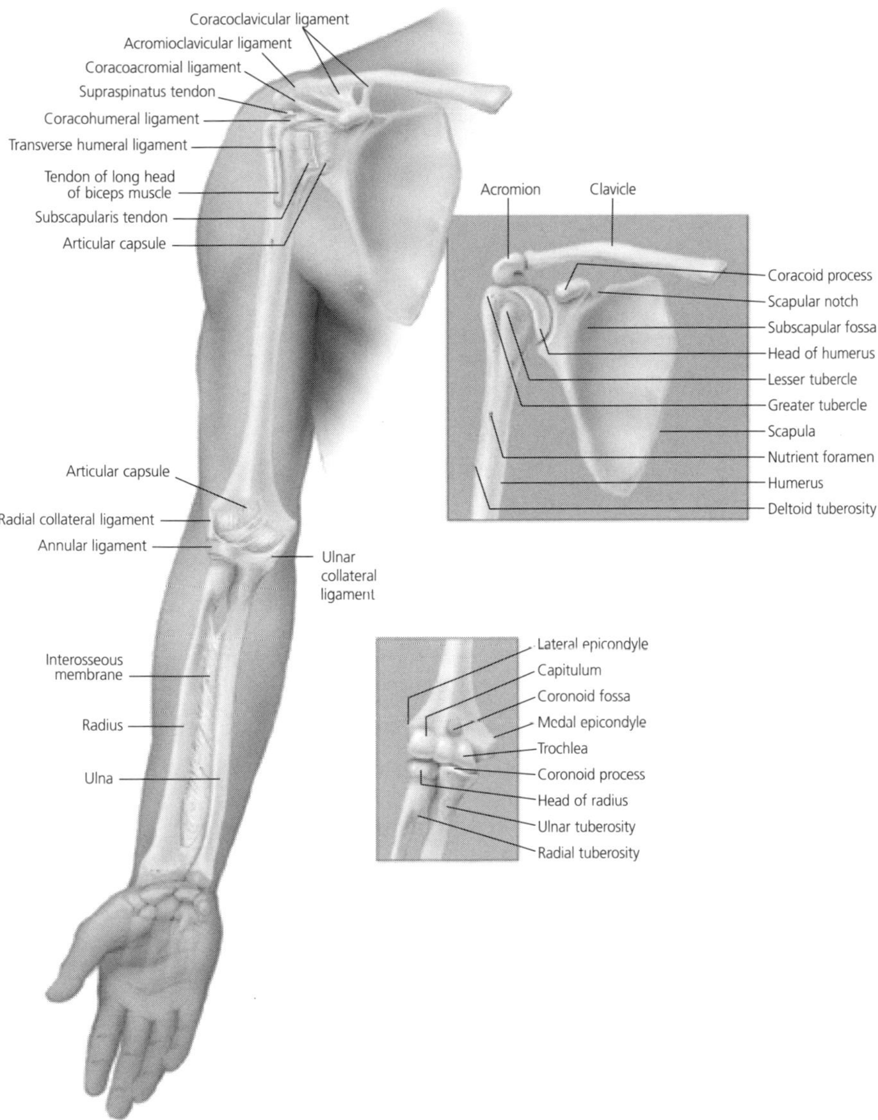

©Scientific Publishing Ltd., Rolling Meadows, IL

PLATE 7. MUSCULAR SYSTEM - HAND AND WRIST

Arthropathies and related disorders

Diffuse diseases of connective tissue	710
Arthropathy associated with infections	711
Crystal arthropathies	712
Arthropathy associated with other disorders classified elsewhere	713
Rheumatoid arthritis and other inflammatory polyarthropathies	714
Osteoarthrosis and allied disorders	715
Other and unspecified arthropathies	716
Other derangement of joint	718
Other and unspecified disorder of joint	719

Rheumatism, excluding the back

Polymyalgia rheumatica	725
Peripheral enthesopathies and allied syndromes	726
Other disorders of synovium, tendon, and bursa	727
Disorders of muscle, ligament, and fascia	728
Other disorders of soft tissues	729

Osteopathies, chondropathies, and acquired musculoskeletal deformities

Osteomyelitis, periostitis, and other infections involving bone	730
Osteitis deformans and osteopathies associated with other disorders classified elsewhere	731
Osteochondropathies	732
Other disorders of bone and cartilage	733
Other acquired deformities of limbs	736
Other acquired deformity	738
Nonallopathic lesions, not elsewhere classified	739

Symptoms, signs and ill-defined conditions 780-799

Sprains and strains of joints and adjacent muscles

Sprains and strains of wrist and hand	842
Other and ill-defined sprains and strains	848

Hand and Wrist

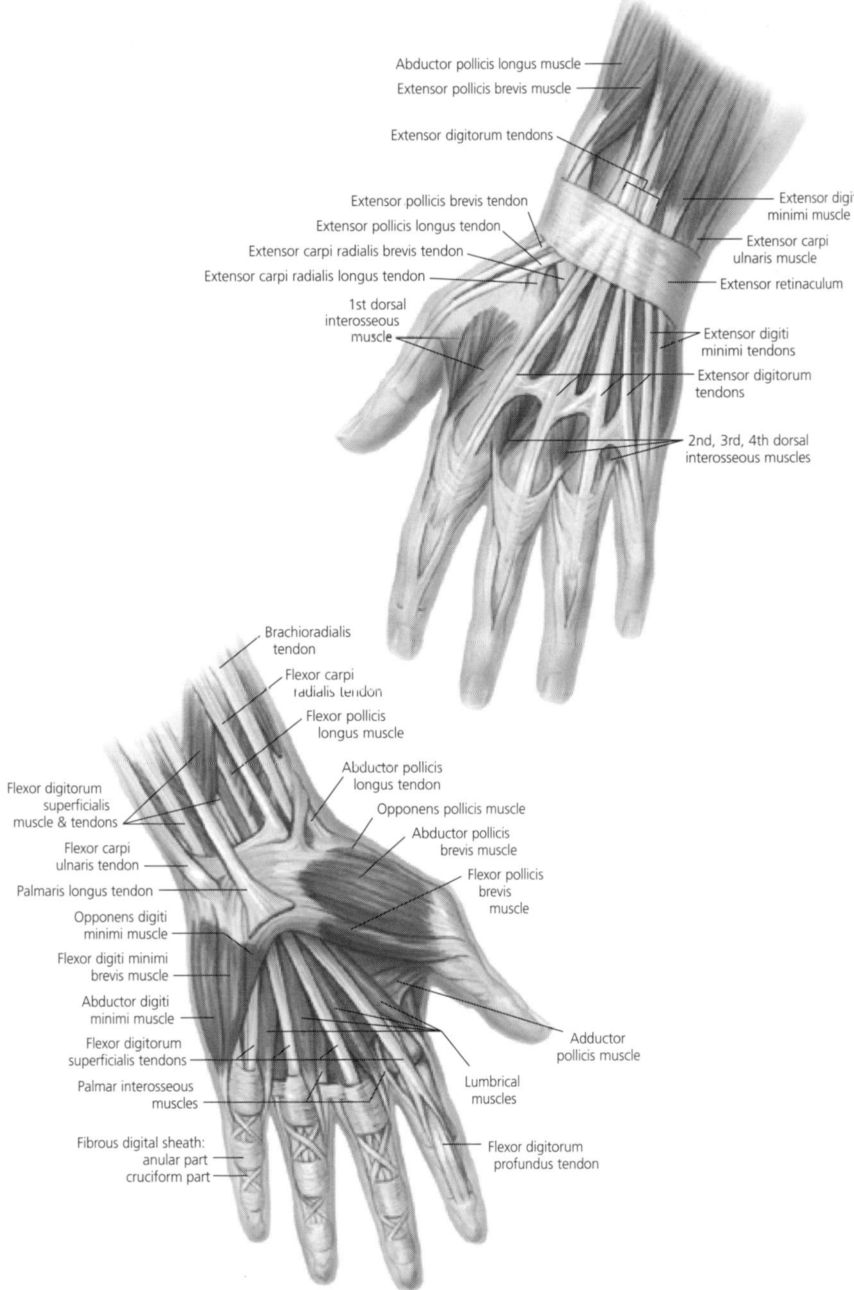

©Practice Management Information Corp., Los Angeles, CA

PLATE 8. MUSCULOSKELETAL SYSTEM - HIP AND KNEE

Arthropathies and related disorders

Diffuse diseases of connective tissue	710
Arthropathy associated with infections	711
Crystal arthropathies	712
Arthropathy associated with other disorders classified elsewhere	713
Rheumatoid arthritis and other inflammatory polyarthropathies	714
Osteoarthrosis and allied disorders	715
Other and unspecified arthropathies	716
Internal derangement of knee	717
Other derangement of joint	718
Other and unspecified disorder of joint	719

Rheumatism, excluding the back

Polymyalgia rheumatica	725
Peripheral enthesopathies and allied syndromes	726
Other disorders of synovium, tendon, and bursa	727
Disorders of muscle, ligament, and fascia	728
Other disorders of soft tissues	729

Osteopathies, chondropathies, and acquired musculoskeletal deformities

Osteomyelitis, periostitis, and other infections involving bone	730
Osteitis deformans and osteopathies associated with other disorders classified elsewhere	731
Osteochondropathies	732
Other disorders of bone and cartilage	733
Other acquired deformities of limbs	736
Curvature of spine	737
Other acquired deformity	738
Nonallopathic lesions, not elsewhere classified	739

Symptoms, signs and ill-defined conditions 780-799

Sprains and strains of joints and adjacent muscles

Sprains and strains of hip and thigh	843
Sprains and strains of knee and leg	844
Other and ill-defined sprains and strains	848

Hip and Knee
(Anterior View)

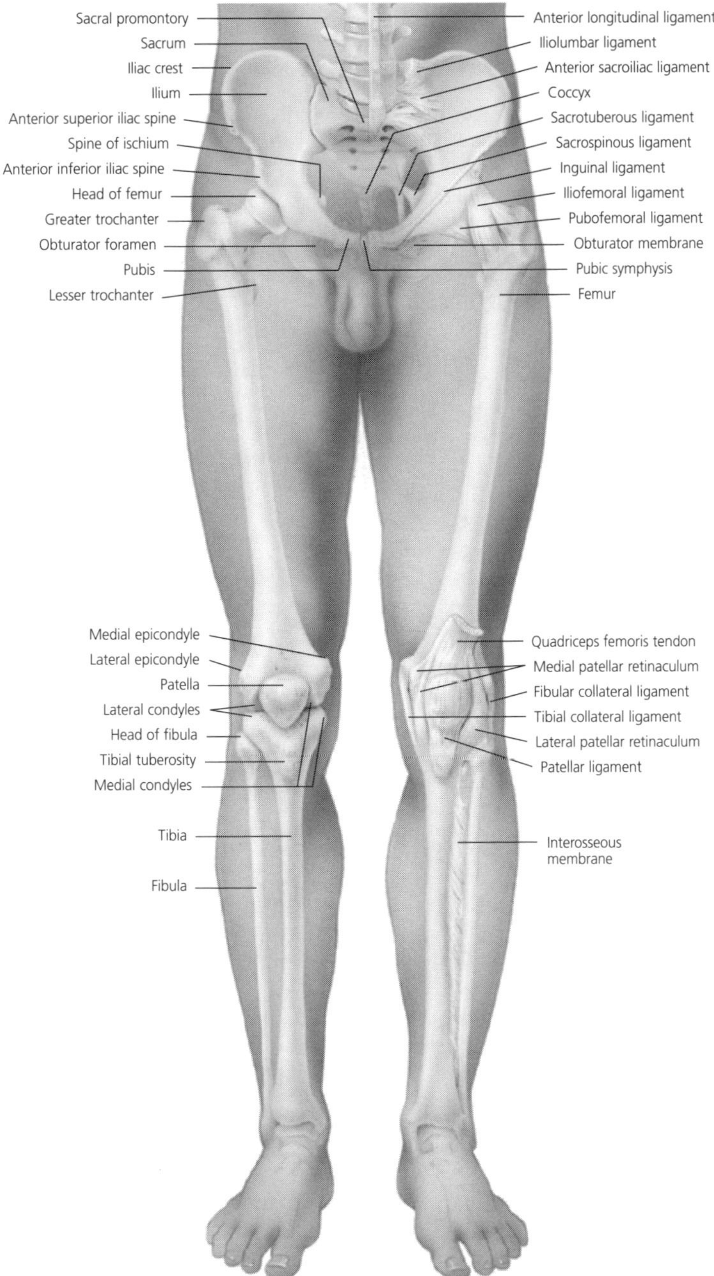

©Scientific Publishing Ltd., Rolling Meadows, IL

PLATE 9. MUSCULOSKELETAL SYSTEM - FOOT AND ANKLE

Arthropathies and related disorders

Diffuse diseases of connective tissue	710
Arthropathy associated with infections	711
Crystal arthropathies	712
Arthropathy associated with other disorders classified elsewhere	713
Rheumatoid arthritis and other inflammatory polyarthropathies	714
Osteoarthrosis and allied disorders	715
Other and unspecified arthropathies	716
Other derangement of joint	718
Other and unspecified disorder of joint	719

Rheumatism, excluding the back

Polymyalgia rheumatica	725
Peripheral enthesopathies and allied syndromes	726
Other disorders of synovium, tendon, and bursa	727
Disorders of muscle, ligament, and fascia	728
Other disorders of soft tissues	729

Osteopathies, chondropathies, and acquired musculoskeletal deformities

Osteomyelitis, periostitis, and other infections involving bone	730
Osteitis deformans and osteopathies associated with other disorders classified elsewhere	731
Osteochondropathies	732
Other disorders of bone and cartilage	733
Flat foot	734
Acquired deformities of toe	735
Other acquired deformities of limbs	736
Other acquired deformity	738
Nonallopathic lesions, not elsewhere classified	739

Symptoms, signs and ill-defined conditions 780-799

Sprains and strains of joints and adjacent muscles

Sprains and strains of ankle and foot	845
Other and ill-defined sprains and strains	848

Foot and Ankle

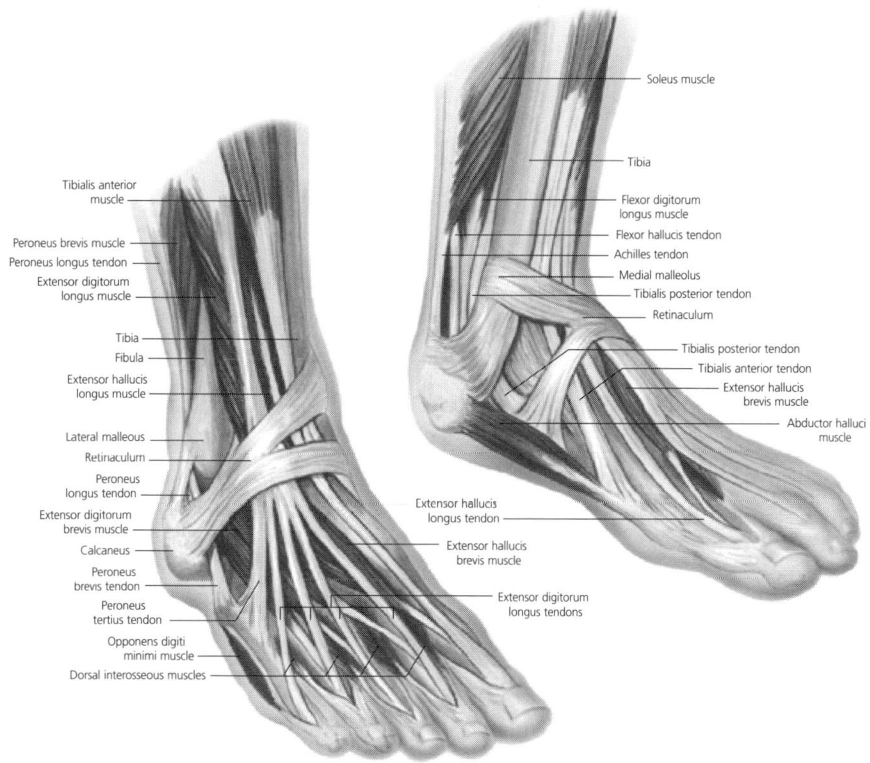

©Practice Management Information Corp., Los Angeles, CA

PLATE 10. SKELETAL SYSTEM - ANTERIOR VIEW

Symptoms, signs and ill-defined conditions 780-799

Fracture of skull

Fracture of vault of skull 800
Fracture of base of skull 801
Fracture of face bones 802
Multiple fractures involving skull or face with other bones 804

Fracture of neck and trunk

Fracture of vertebral column without mention of spinal cord injury 805
Fracture of vertebral column with spinal cord injury 806
Fracture of rib
Fracture of pelvis 808

Fracture of upper limb

Fracture of clavicle 810
Fracture of scapula 811
Fracture of humerus 812
Fracture of radius and ulna 813
Fracture of carpal bone(s) 814
Fracture of metacarpal bone(s) 815
Fracture of one or more phalanges of hand 816
Multiple fractures of hand bones 817

Fracture of lower limb

Fracture of neck of femur 820
Fracture of other and unspecified parts of femur 821
Fracture of patella 822
Fracture of tibia and fibula 823
Fracture of ankle 824
Fracture of one or more tarsal and metatarsal bones 825
Fracture of one or more phalanges of foot 826

Dislocation

Dislocation of jaw 830
Dislocation of shoulder 831
Dislocation of elbow 832
Dislocation of wrist 833
Dislocation of finger 834
Dislocation of hip 835
Dislocation of knee 836
Dislocation of ankle 837
Dislocation of foot 838

Skeletal System
(Anterior View)

Frontal bone
Temporal bone
Nasal conchae
Maxilla
Manubrium of sternum
Coracoid process
Acromion
Greater tubercle
Head of humerus
Scapula
Humerus
True ribs (1–7)
False ribs (8–12)
Medial epicondyle
Lateral epicondyle
Radius
Ulna
Sacrum
Anterior superior iliac spine
Head of femur
Greater trochanter
Parietal bone
Orbit
Zygomatic bone
Nasal septum
Mandible
Hyoid bone
Clavicle
Coracoclavicular ligament
Supraspinatus tendon
Subscapularis tendon
Body of sternum
Xiphoid process
Costal cartilages
Anterior longitudinal ligament
Ulnar collateral ligament
Radial collateral ligament
Annular ligament
L3
Iliac crest
Anterior sacroiliac ligament
Interosseous membrane
Inguinal ligament
Coccyx
Iliofemoral ligament
Pubic symphysis
Metacarpals
Proximal phalanges
Middle phalanges
Distal phalanges
Femur
Medial epicondyle
Lateral epicondyle
Patella
Head of fibula
Tibial tuberosity
Quadriceps femoris tendon
Tibial collateral ligament
Fibular collateral ligament
Patellar ligament
Tibia
Fibula
Interosseous membrane
Medial malleolus
Lateral malleolus

Key to Carpal Bones

- **A** Scaphoid
- **B** Trapezium
- **C** Trapezoid
- **D** Capitate
- **E** Lunate
- **F** Pisiform
- **G** Triquetral
- **H** Hamate

Key to Tarsal Bones

- **J** Intermediate cuneiform
- **K** Lateral cuneiform
- **L** Cuboid
- **M** Talus
- **N** Navicular
- **O** Calcaneus
- **P** Medial cuneiform

©Scientific Publishing Ltd., Rolling Meadows, IL

PLATE 11. SKELETAL SYSTEM - POSTERIOR VIEW

Symptoms, signs and ill-defined conditions 780-799

Fracture of skull

Fracture of vault of skull 800
Fracture of base of skull 801
Fracture of face bones 802
Multiple fractures involving skull or face with other bones 804

Fracture of neck and trunk

Fracture of vertebral column without mention of spinal cord injury 805
Fracture of vertebral column with spinal cord injury 806
Fracture of rib
Fracture of pelvis 808

Fracture of upper limb

Fracture of clavicle 810
Fracture of scapula 811
Fracture of humerus 812
Fracture of radius and ulna 813
Fracture of carpal bone(s) 814
Fracture of metacarpal bone(s) 815
Fracture of one or more phalanges of hand 816
Multiple fractures of hand bones 817

Fracture of lower limb

Fracture of neck of femur 820
Fracture of other and unspecified parts of femur 821
Fracture of patella 822
Fracture of tibia and fibula 823
Fracture of ankle 824
Fracture of one or more tarsal and metatarsal bones 825
Fracture of one or more phalanges of foot 826

Dislocation

Dislocation of jaw 830
Dislocation of shoulder 831
Dislocation of elbow 832
Dislocation of wrist 833
Dislocation of finger 834
Dislocation of hip 835
Dislocation of knee 836
Dislocation of ankle 837
Dislocation of foot 838

Skeletal System
(Posterior View)

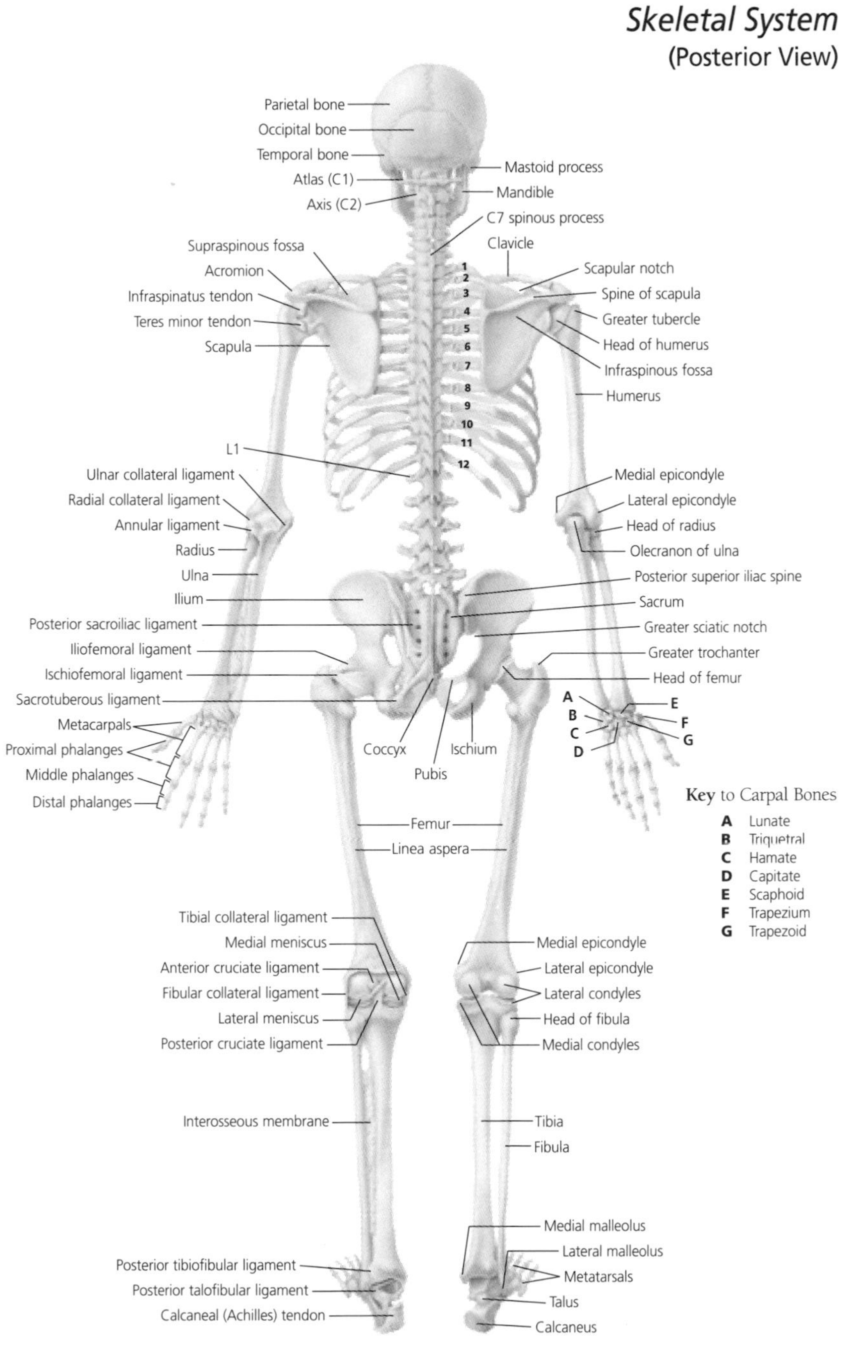

Key to Carpal Bones

A Lunate
B Triquetral
C Hamate
D Capitate
E Scaphoid
F Trapezium
G Trapezoid

©Scientific Publishing Ltd., Rolling Meadows, IL

PLATE 12. SKELETAL SYSTEM - VERTEBRAL COLUMN

Arthropathies and related disorders

Diffuse diseases of connective tissue	710
Arthropathy associated with infections	711
Crystal arthropathies	712
Arthropathy associated with other disorders classified elsewhere	713
Rheumatoid arthritis and other inflammatory polyarthropathies	714
Osteoarthrosis and allied disorders	715

Dorsopathies

Ankylosing spondylitis and other inflammatory spondylopathies	720
Spondylosis and allied disorders	721
Intervertebral disc disorders	722
Other disorders of cervical region	723
Other and unspecified disorders of back	724

Osteopathies, chondropathies, and acquired musculoskeletal deformities

Osteomyelitis, periostitis, and other infections involving bone	730
Osteitis deformans and osteopathies associated with other disorders classified elsewhere	731
Osteochondropathies	732
Other disorders of bone and cartilage	733
Curvature of spine	737
Other acquired deformity	738
Nonallopathic lesions, not elsewhere classified	739

Symptoms, signs and ill-defined conditions — 780-799

Fracture of neck and trunk

Fracture of vertebral column without mention of spinal cord injury	805
Fracture of vertebral column with spinal cord injury	806

Vertebral Column
(Lateral View)

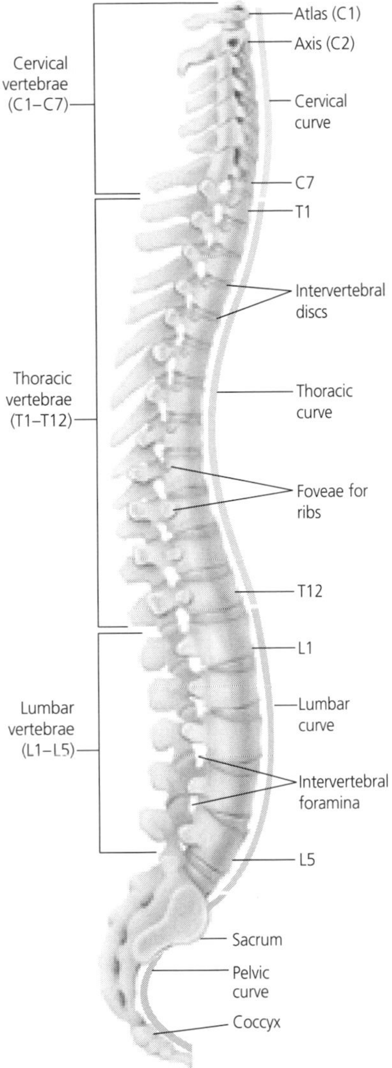

©Scientific Publishing Ltd., Rolling Meadows, IL

PLATE 13. RESPIRATORY SYSTEM

Neoplasms

Malignant neoplasm of respiratory and intrathoracic organs	160-165
Malignant neoplasm of larynx	161
Malignant neoplasm of trachea, bronchus, and lung	162
Benign neoplasm of respiratory and intrathoracic organs	212
Carcinoma in situ of respiratory system	231

Acute respiratory infections

Acute nasopharyngitis [common cold]	460
Acute sinusitis	461
Acute pharyngitis	462
Acute tonsillitis	463
Acute laryngitis and tracheitis	464
Acute upper respiratory infections of multiple or unspecified sites	465
Acute bronchitis and bronchiolitis	466

Other diseases of upper respiratory tract

Deviated nasal septum	470
Nasal polyps	471
Chronic pharyngitis and nasopharyngitis	472
Chronic sinusitis	473
Chronic disease of tonsils and adenoids	474
Peritonsillar abscess	475
Chronic laryngitis and laryngotracheitis	476
Allergic rhinitis	477

Pneumonia and influenza

Viral pneumonia	480
Pneumococcal pneumonia [Streptococcus pneumoniae pneumonia]	481
Influenza	487

Chronic obstructive pulmonary disease and allied conditions

Chronic bronchitis	491
Emphysema	492
Asthma	493
Bronchiectasis	494
Extrinsic allergic alveolitis	495

Other diseases of respiratory system

Empyema	510
Pleurisy	511
Pneumothorax	512
Abscess of lung and mediastinum	513
Pulmonary congestion and hypostasis	514
Postinflammatory pulmonary fibrosis	515

Respiratory System

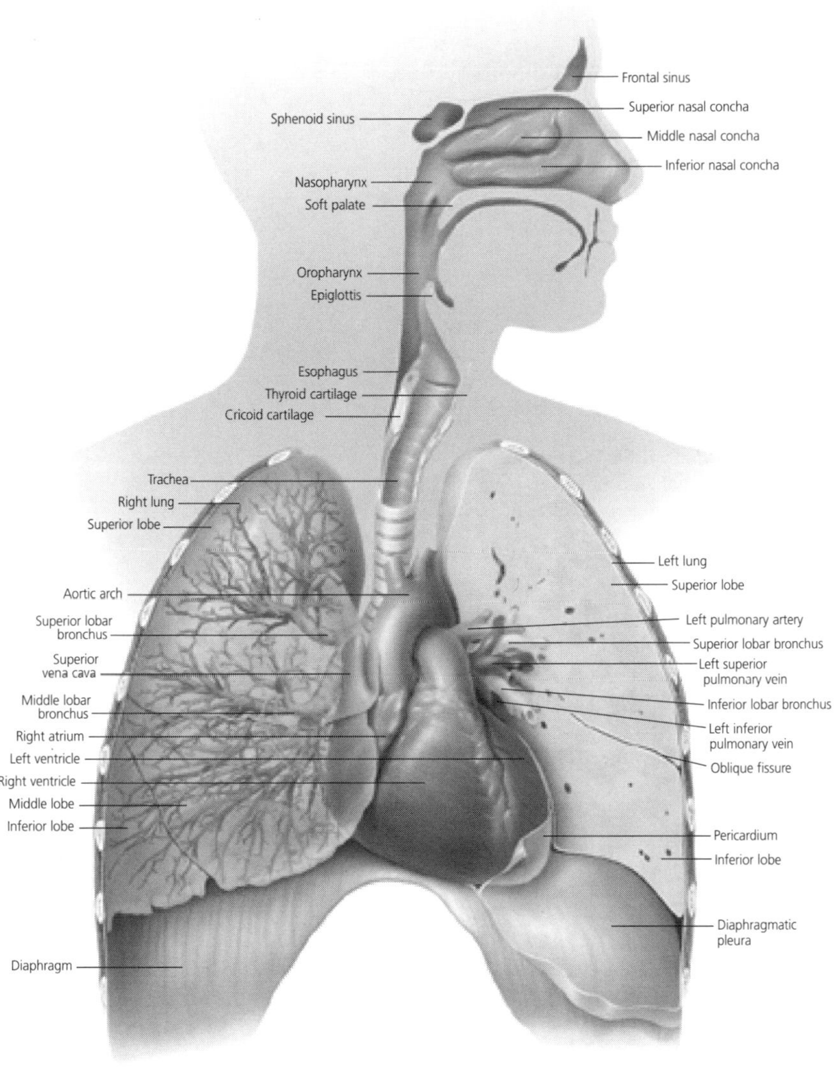

©Scientific Publishing Ltd., Rolling Meadows, IL

PLATE 14. HEART AND PERICARDIUM

Acute rheumatic fever

Rheumatic fever without mention of heart involvement	390
Rheumatic fever with heart involvement	391
Rheumatic chorea	392

Chronic rheumatic heart disease

Chronic rheumatic pericarditis	393
Diseases of mitral valve	394
Diseases of aortic valve	395
Diseases of mitral and aortic valves	396
Diseases of other endocardial structures	397

Hypertensive disease

Essential hypertension	401
Hypertensive heart disease	402
Hypertensive renal disease	403
Hypertensive heart and renal disease	404
Secondary hypertension	405

Ischemic heart disease

Acute myocardial infarction	410
Other acute and subacute form of ischemic heart disease	411
Old myocardial infarction	412
Angina pectoris	413

Diseases of pulmonary circulation

Acute pulmonary heart disease	415
Chronic pulmonary heart disease	416
Other diseases of pulmonary circulation	417

Other forms of heart disease

Acute pericarditis	420
Acute and subacute endocarditis	421
Acute myocarditis	422
Other diseases of pericardium	423
Other diseases of endocardium	424
Cardiomyopathy	425
Conduction disorders	426
Cardiac dysrhythmias	427
Heart failure	428

Symptoms, signs and ill-defined conditions 780-799

Heart
(External View)

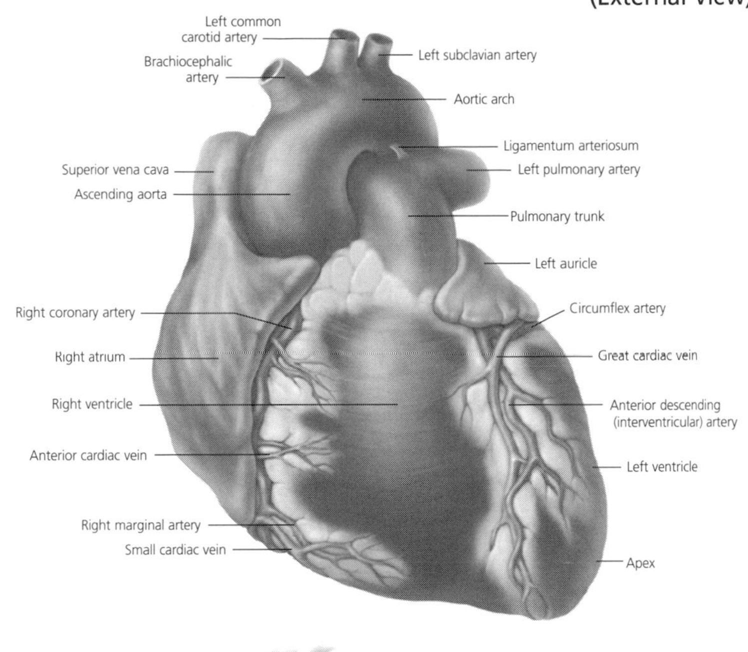

Heart
(Internal View)

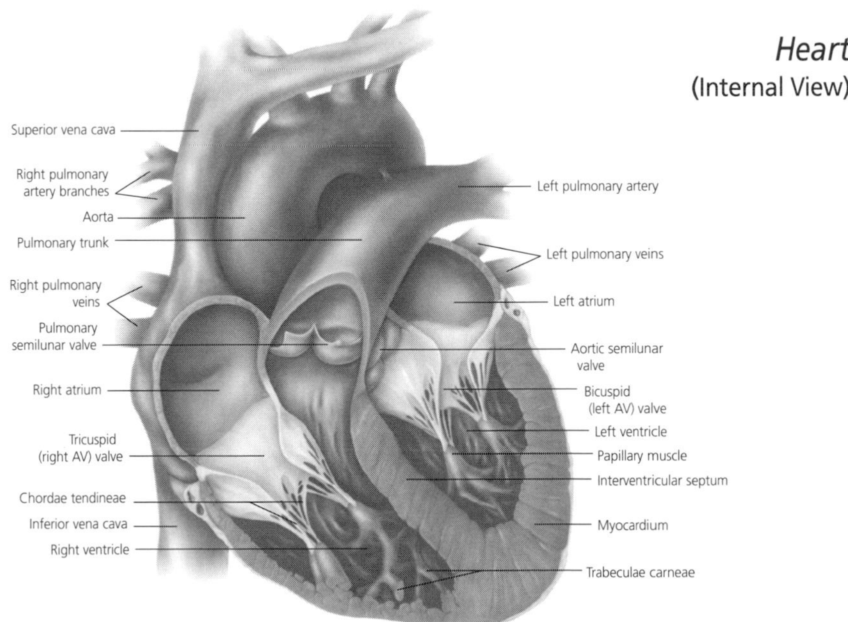

©Scientific Publishing Ltd., Rolling Meadows, IL

PLATE 15. CIRCULATORY SYSTEM

Diseases of arteries, arterioles, and capillaries

Atherosclerosis	440
Aortic aneurysm and dissection	441
Arterial embolism and thrombosis	444
Polyarteritis nodosa and allied conditions	446
Other disorders of arteries and arterioles	447
Diseases of capillaries	448

Diseases of veins and lymphatics, and other circulatory system

Phlebitis and thrombophlebitis	451
Portal vein thrombosis	452
Varicose veins of lower extremities	454
Hemorrhoids	455
Varicose veins of other sites	456
Noninfective disorders of lymphatic channels	457
Hypotension	458

Symptoms, signs and ill-defined conditions 780-799

Injury to blood vessels

Injury to blood vessels of head and neck	900
Injury to blood vessels of thorax	901
Injury to blood vessels of abdomen and pelvis	902
Injury to blood vessels of upper extremity	903
Injury to blood vessels of lower extremity and unspecified sites	904

Vascular System

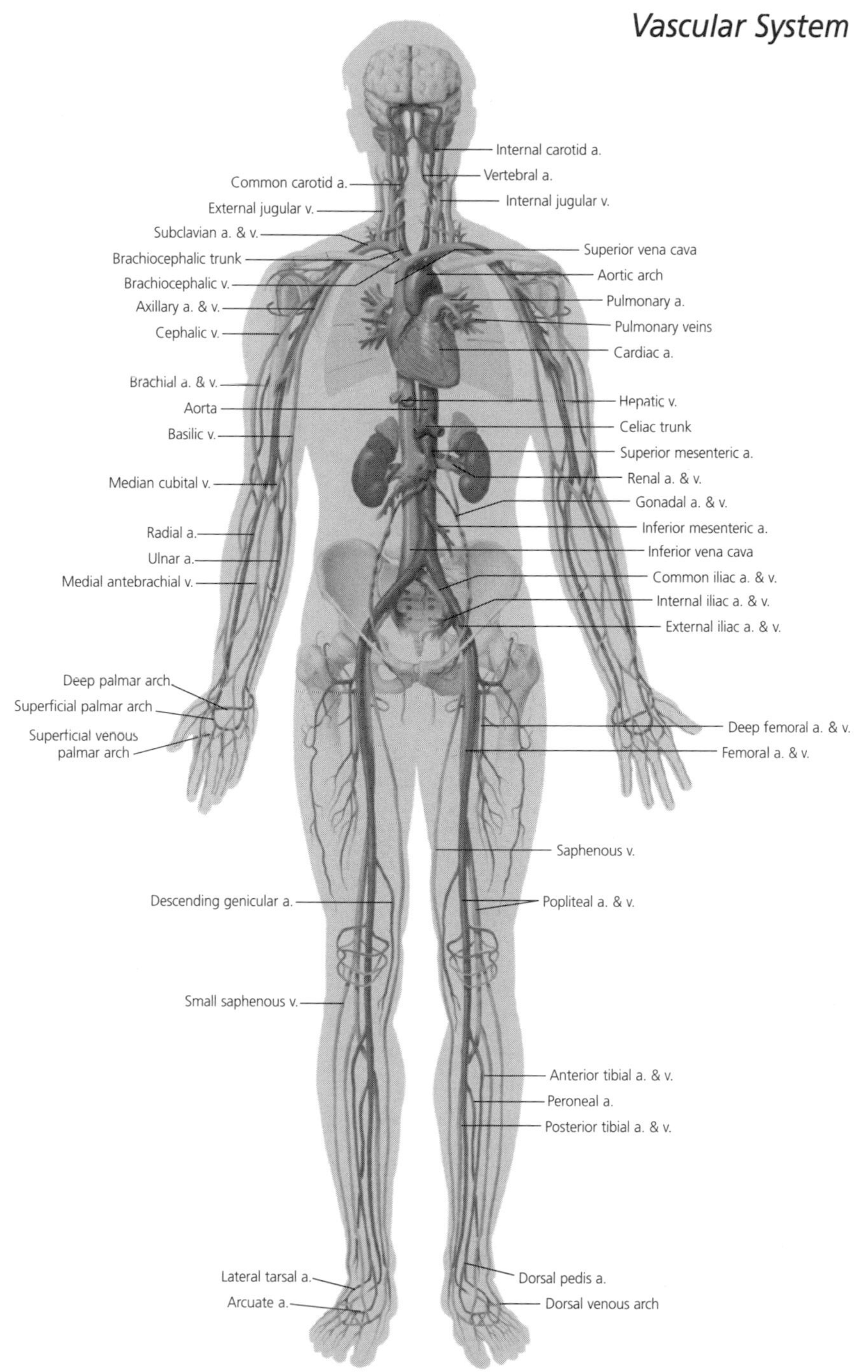

©Practice Management Information Corp., Los Angeles, CA

PLATE 16. DIGESTIVE SYSTEM

Malignant neoplasms of digestive organs and peritoneum

Malignant neoplasm of esophagus	150
Malignant neoplasm of stomach	151
Malignant neoplasm of small intestine, including duodenum	152
Malignant neoplasm of colon	153
Malignant neoplasm of rectum, rectosigmoid junction, and anus	154
Malignant neoplasm of liver and intrahepatic bile ducts	155
Malignant neoplasm of gallbladder and extrahepatic bile ducts	156
Malignant neoplasm of pancreas	157
Benign neoplasm of other parts of digestive system	211
Carcinoma in situ of digestive organs	230

Diseases of esophagus, stomach, and duodenum

Diseases of esophagus	530
Gastric ulcer	531
Duodenal ulcer	532
Gastrojejunal ulcer	534
Gastritis and duodenitis	535

Appendicitis

Acute appendicitis	540
Appendicitis, unqualified	541

Hernia of abdominal cavity

Inguinal hernia	550
Other hernia of abdominal cavity, with gangrene	551
Other hernia of abdominal cavity, with obstruction, but without mention of gangrene	552
Other hernia of abdominal cavity without mention of obstruction or gangrene	553

Noninfectious enteritis and colitis

Regional enteritis	555
Ulcerative colitis	556
Vascular insufficiency of intestine	557

Other diseases of intestines and peritoneum

Intestinal obstruction without mention of hernia	560
Diverticula of intestine	562
Anal fissure and fistula	565
Abscess of anal and rectal regions	566
Peritonitis	567

Other diseases of digestive system

Acute and subacute necrosis of liver	570
Chronic liver disease and cirrhosis	571
Cholelithiasis	574
Diseases of pancreas	577
Gastrointestinal hemorrhage	578

Digestive System

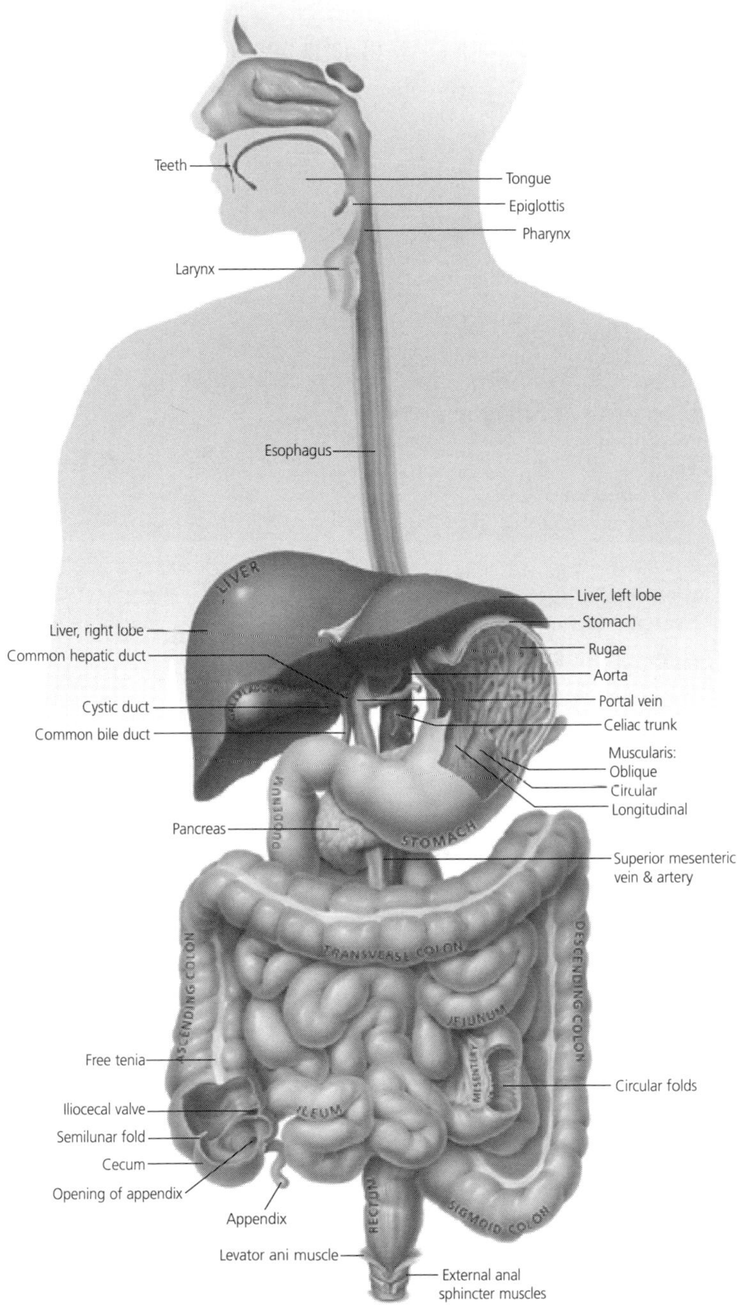

©Practice Management Information Corp., Los Angeles, CA

PLATE 17. GENITOURINARY SYSTEM

Neoplasms

Malignant neoplasm of bladder	188
Malignant neoplasm of kidney and other and unspecified urinary organs	189
Benign neoplasm of kidney and other urinary organs	223

Nephritis, nephrotic syndrome, and nephrosis

Acute glomerulonephritis	580
Nephrotic syndrome	581
Chronic glomerulonephritis	582
Nephritis and nephropathy, not specified as acute or chronic	583
Acute renal failure	584
Chronic renal failure	585
Disorders resulting from impaired renal function	588

Other diseases of urinary system

Infections of kidney	590
Hydronephrosis	591
Calculus of kidney and ureter	592
Calculus of lower urinary tract	594
Cystitis	595
Urethritis, not sexually transmitted, and urethral syndrome	597
Urethral stricture	598

Symptoms, signs and ill-defined conditions 780-799

Urinary System

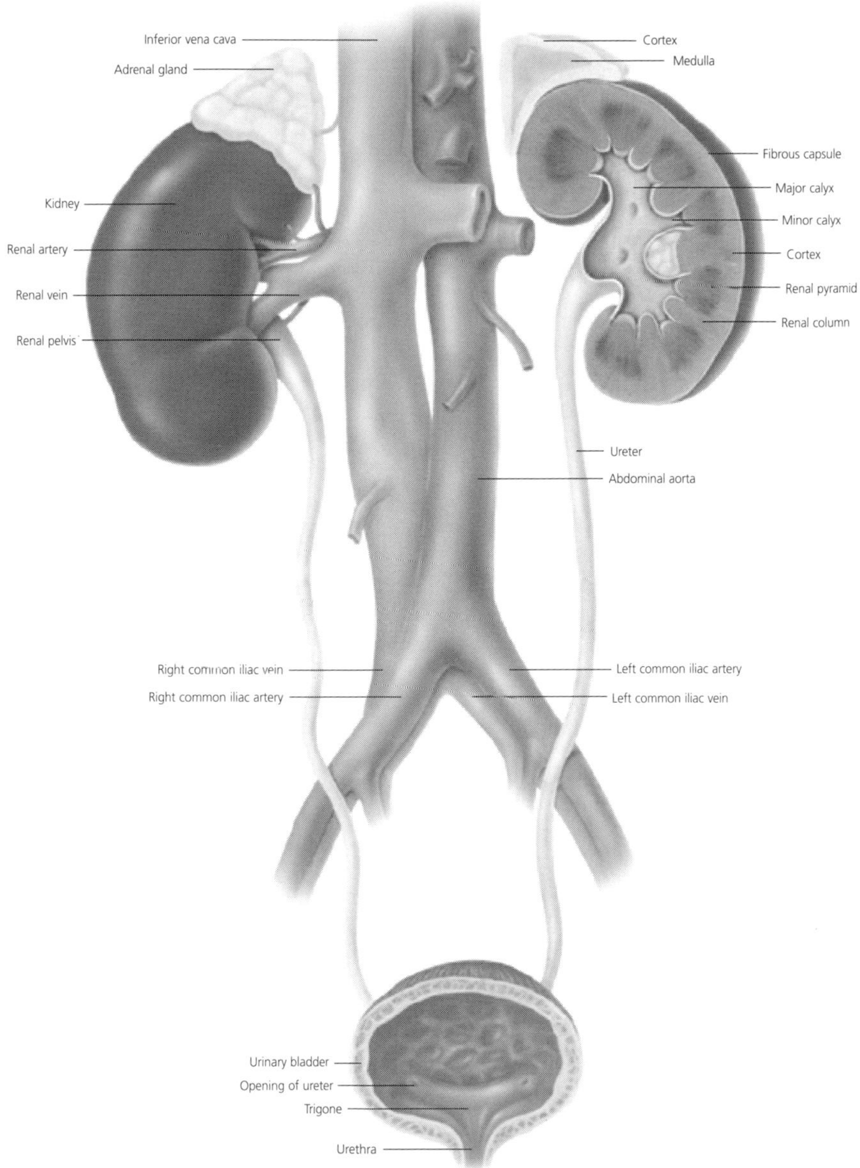

©Practice Management Information Corp., Los Angeles, CA

PLATE 18. MALE GENITAL ORGANS

Neoplasms

Malignant neoplasm of prostate	185
Malignant neoplasm of testis	186
Malignant neoplasm of penis and other male genital organs	187
Benign neoplasm of male genital organs	222

Diseases of male genital organs

Hyperplasia of prostate	600
Inflammatory diseases of prostate	601
Hydrocele	603
Orchitis and epididymitis	604
Redundant prepuce and phimosis	605
Infertility, male	606
Disorders of penis	607

Symptoms, signs and ill-defined conditions 780-799

Male Reproductive System

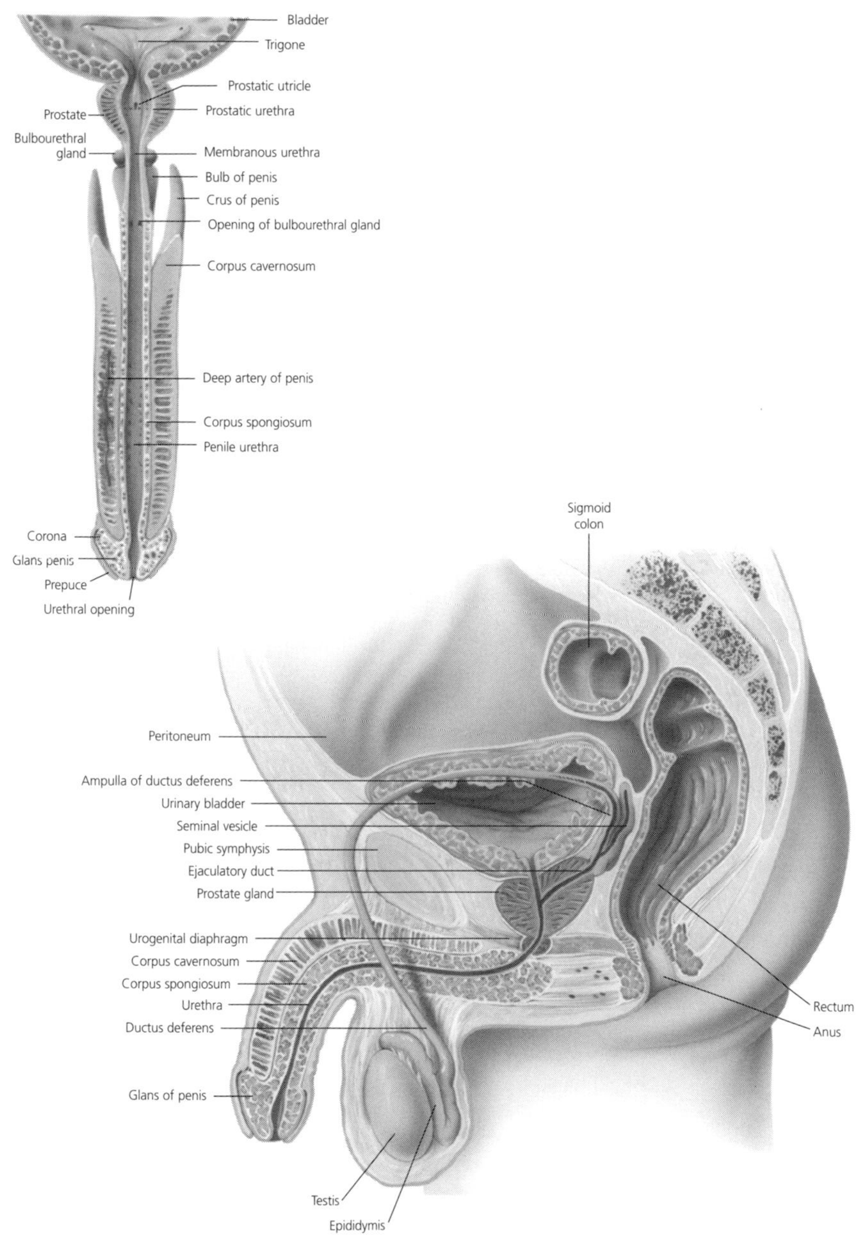

©Practice Management Information Corp., Los Angeles, CA

PLATE 19. FEMALE GENITAL ORGANS

Neoplasms

Malignant neoplasm of uterus, part unspecified	179
Malignant neoplasm of cervix uteri	180
Malignant neoplasm of placenta	181
Malignant neoplasm of body of uterus	182
Malignant neoplasm of ovary and other uterine adnexa	183
Other benign neoplasm of uterus	219
Benign neoplasm of ovary	220
Benign neoplasm of other female genital organs	221

Inflammatory disease of female pelvic organs

Inflammatory disease of ovary, fallopian tube, pelvic cellular tissue, and peritoneum	614
Inflammatory diseases of uterus, except cervix	615
Inflammatory disease of cervix, vagina, and vulva	616

Other disorders of female genital tract

Endometriosis	617
Genital prolapse	618
Fistula involving female genital tract	619
Noninflammatory disorders of ovary, fallopian tube, and broad ligament	620
Disorders of uterus, not elsewhere classified	621
Noninflammatory disorders of cervix	622
Noninflammatory disorders of vagina	623
Noninflammatory disorders of vulva and perineum	624
Pain and other symptoms associated with female genital organs	625
Disorders of menstruation and other abnormal bleeding from female genital tract	626
Menopausal and postmenopausal disorders	627
Infertility, female	628

Symptoms, signs and ill-defined conditions 780-799

Female Reproductive System

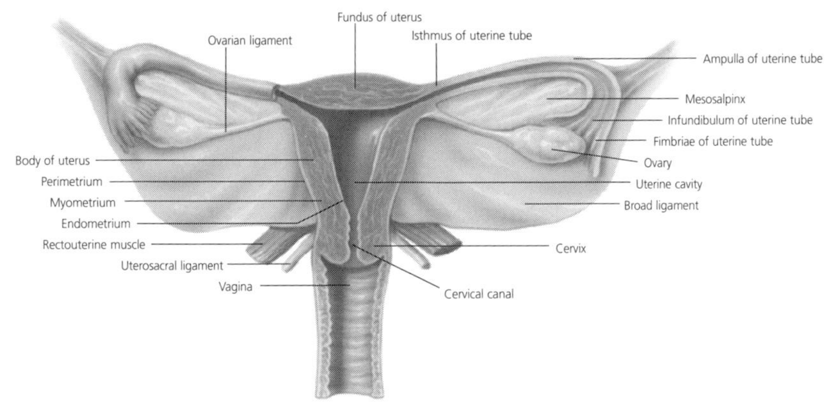

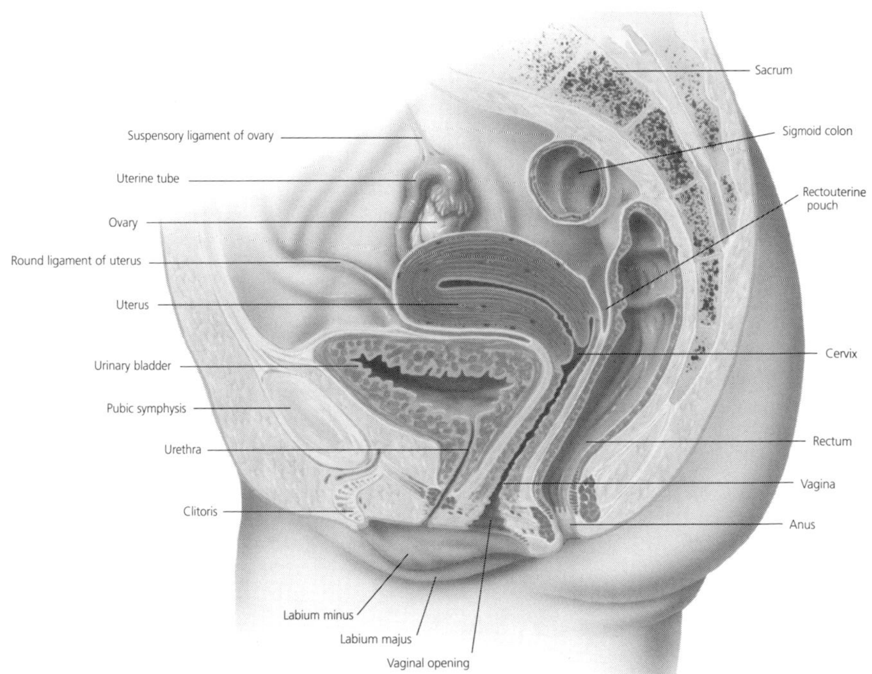

©Practice Management Information Corp., Los Angeles, CA

PLATE 20. PREGNANCY, CHILDBIRTH AND THE PUERPERIUM

Ectopic and molar pregnancy

Hydatidiform mole	630
Other abnormal product of conception	631
Missed abortion	632
Ectopic pregnancy	633

Other pregnancy with abortive outcome

Abortion	634
Legally induced abortion	635
Complications following abortion and ectopic and molar pregnancies	639

Complications mainly related to pregnancy

Hemorrhage in early pregnancy	640
Antepartum hemorrhage, abruptio placentae, and placenta previa	641
Hypertension complicating pregnancy, childbirth, and the puerperium	642
Excessive vomiting in pregnancy	643
Early or threatened labor	644
Prolonged pregnancy	645

Normal delivery, other indications for care in pregnancy and delivery

Normal delivery	650
Multiple gestation	651
Malposition and malpresentation of fetus	652
Disproportion	653
Polyhydramnios	657

Complications occurring mainly in the course of labor and delivery

Obstructed labor	660
Abnormality of forces of labor	661
Long labor	662
Umbilical cord complications	663
Trauma to perineum and vulva during delivery	664
Postpartum hemorrhage	666
Retained placenta or membranes, without hemorrhage	667

Complications of the puerperium

Major puerperal infection	670
Venous complications in pregnancy and the puerperium	671
Pyrexia of unknown origin during the puerperium	672
Obstetrical pulmonary embolism	673

Persons Encountering Health Services in Circumstances Related to Reproduction

Normal pregnancy	V22
Supervision of high-risk pregnancy	V23
Postpartum care and examination	V24
Encounter for contraceptive management	V25
Procreative management	V26

Female Reproductive System: Pregnancy
(Lateral View)

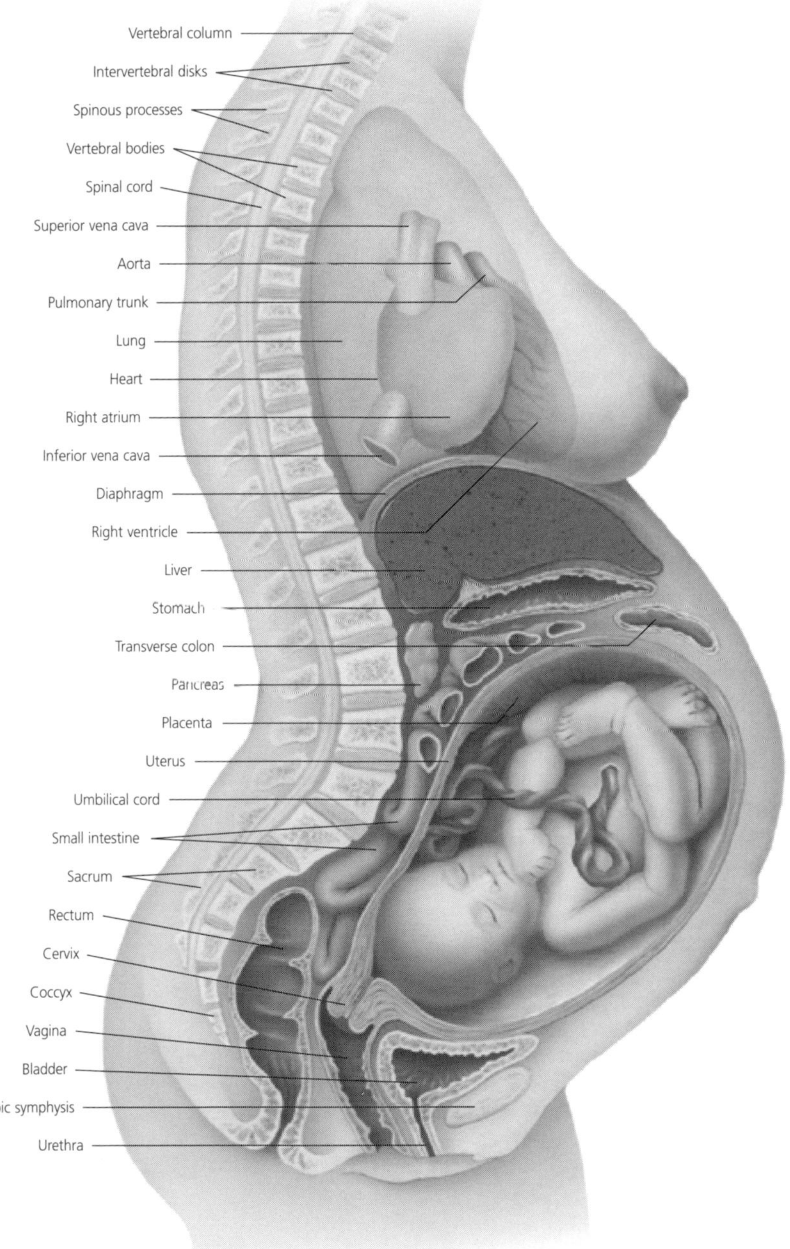

©Practice Management Information Corp., Los Angeles, CA

PLATE 21. NERVOUS SYSTEM - BRAIN

Neoplasms

Malignant neoplasm of brain	191

Organic psychotic conditions

Senile and presenile organic psychotic conditions	290
Alcoholic psychoses	291
Drug psychoses	292
Transient organic psychotic conditions	293
Other organic psychotic conditions	

Other psychoses

Schizophrenic psychoses	295
Affective psychoses	296
Paranoid states	
Other nonorganic psychoses	298
Psychoses with origin specific to childhood	299

Neurotic, personality, and other nonpsychotic disorders

Neurotic disorders	300
Personality disorders	301
Specific nonpsychotic mental disorders due to organic brain damage	310
Hyperkinetic syndrome of childhood	314

Mental retardation

Mild mental retardation	317
Other specified mental retardation	318
Unspecified mental retardation	319

Cerebrovascular disease

Subarachnoid hemorrhage	430
Intracerebral hemorrhage	431
Occlusion and stenosis of precerebral arteries	433
Occlusion of cerebral arteries	434
Transient cerebral ischemia	435
Acute but ill-defined cerebrovascular disease	436
Late effects of cerebrovascular disease	438

Intracranial injury, excluding those with skull fracture

Concussion	850
Cerebral laceration and contusion	851
Subarachnoid, subdural, and extradural hemorrhage, following injury	852
Intracranial injury of other and unspecified nature	854

Symptoms, signs and ill-defined conditions 780-799

Brain
(Base View)

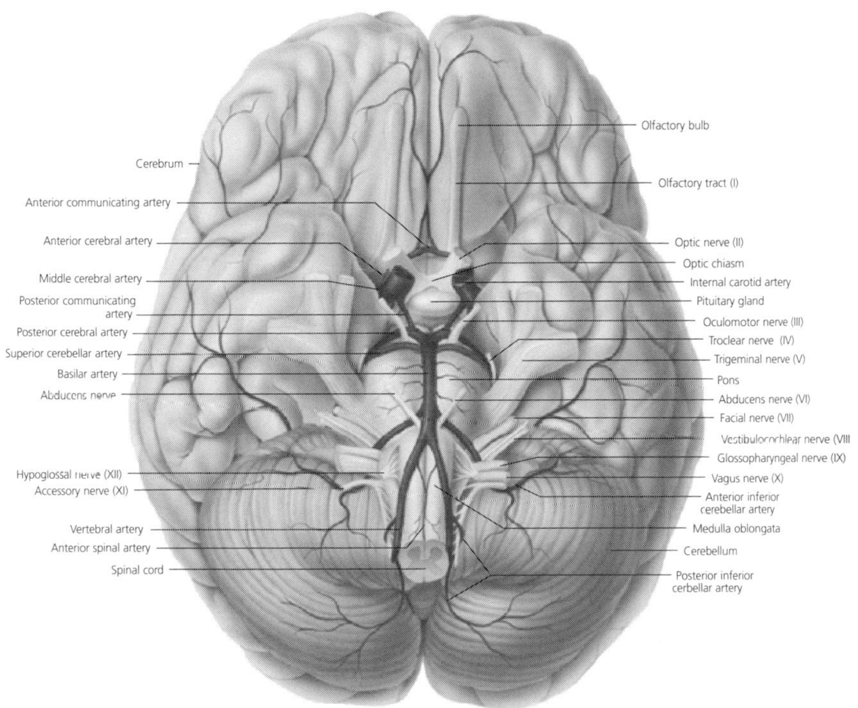

©Practice Management Information Corp., Los Angeles, CA

PLATE 22. NERVOUS SYSTEM

Inflammatory diseases of the central nervous system

Bacterial meningitis	320
Meningitis due to other organisms	321
Encephalitis, myelitis, and encephalomyelitis	323
Intracranial and intraspinal abscess	324
Phlebitis and thrombophlebitis of intracranial venous sinuses	325
Late effects of intracranial abscess or pyogenic infection	326

Hereditary and degenerative diseases of the central nervous system

Cerebral degenerations usually manifest in childhood	330
Other cerebral degenerations	331
Parkinson's disease	332
Spinocerebellar disease	334
Anterior horn cell disease	335
Other diseases of spinal cord	336
Disorders of the autonomic nervous system	337

Other disorders of the central nervous system

Multiple sclerosis	340
Other demyelinating diseases of central nervous system	341
Hemiplegia and hemiparesis	342
Infantile cerebral palsy	343
Other paralytic syndromes	344
Epilepsy	345
Migraine	346
Cataplexy and narcolepsy	347

Disorders of the peripheral nervous system

Trigeminal nerve disorders	350
Facial nerve disorders	351
Disorders of other cranial nerves	352
Nerve root and plexus disorders	353
Mononeuritis of upper limb and mononeuritis multiplex	354
Mononeuritis of lower limb and unspecified site	355
Hereditary and idiopathic peripheral neuropathy	356
Inflammatory and toxic neuropathy	357
Myoneural disorders	358
Muscular dystrophies and other myopathies	359

Injury to nerves and spinal cord

Injury to optic nerve and pathways	950
Injury to other cranial nerve(s)	951
Spinal cord injury without evidence of spinal bone injury	952
Injury to nerve roots and spinal plexus	953
Injury to other nerve(s) of trunk excluding shoulder and pelvic girdles	954
Injury to peripheral nerve(s) of shoulder girdle and upper limb	955
Injury to peripheral nerve(s) of pelvic girdle and lower limb	956

Nervous System

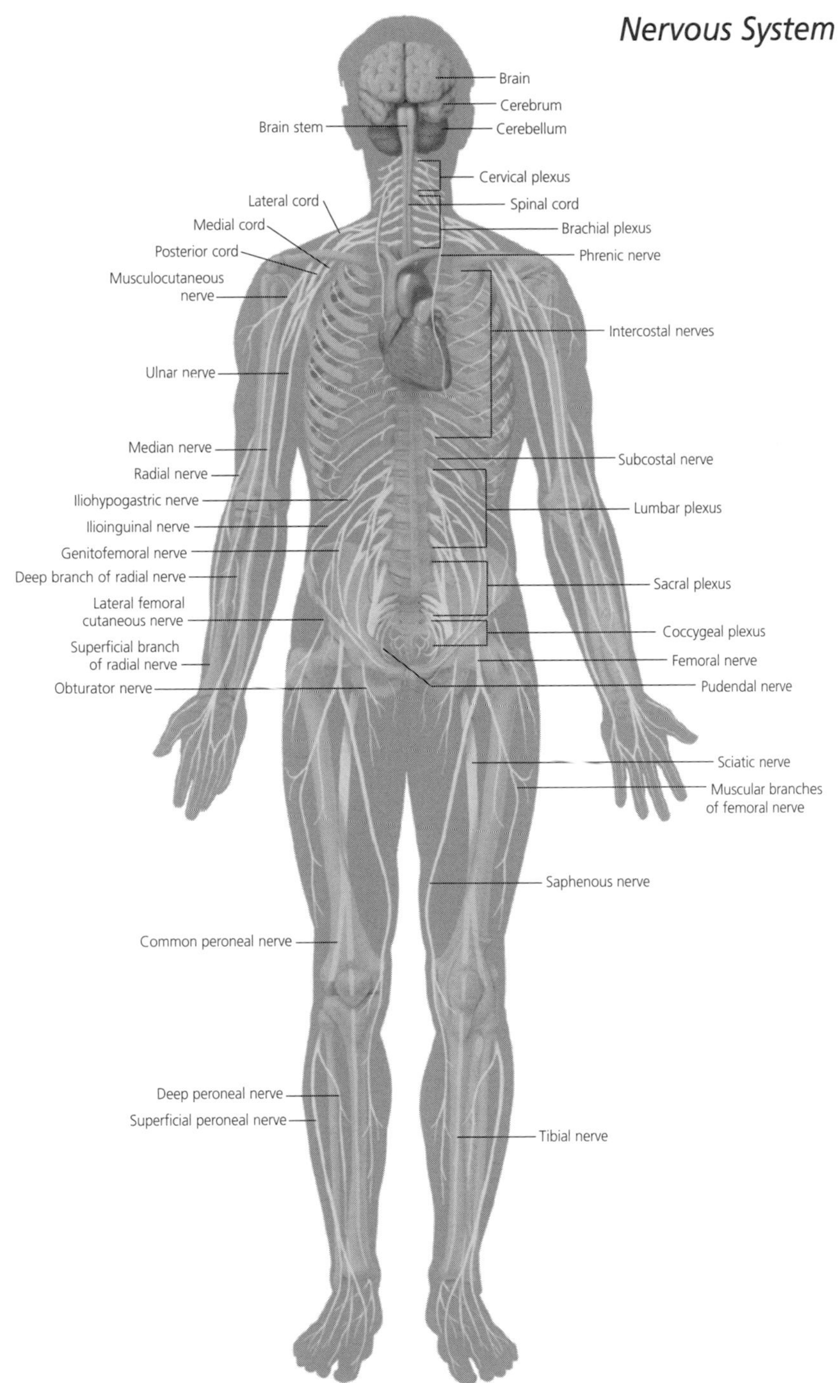

©Practice Management Information Corp., Los Angeles, CA

PLATE 23. EYE AND OCULAR ADNEXA

Disorders of the eye and adnexa

Disorders of the globe	360
Retinal detachments and defects	361
Other retinal disorders	362
Chorioretinal inflammations and scars and other disorders of choroid	363
Disorders of iris and ciliary body	364
Glaucoma	365
Cataract	366
Disorders of refraction and accommodation	367
Visual disturbances	368
Blindness and low vision	369
Keratitis	370
Corneal opacity and other disorders of cornea	371
Disorders of conjunctiva	372
Inflammation of eyelids	373
Other disorders of eyelids	374
Disorders of lacrimal system	375
Disorders of the orbit	376
Disorders of optic nerve and visual pathways	377
Strabismus and other disorders of binocular eye movements	378

Symptoms, signs and ill-defined conditions 780-799

Right Eye
(Horizontal Section)

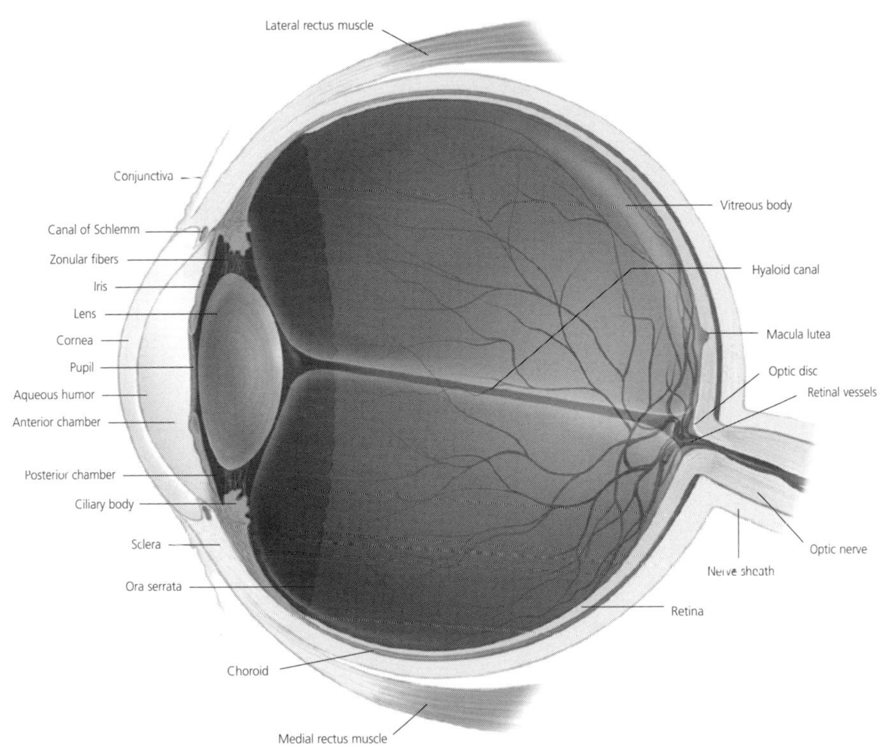

©Scientific Publishing Ltd., Rolling Meadows, IL

PLATE 24. AUDITORY SYSTEM

Diseases of the ear and mastoid process

Disorders of external ear	380
Nonsuppurative otitis media and Eustachian tube disorders	381
Suppurative and unspecified otitis media	382
Mastoiditis and related conditions	383
Other disorders of tympanic membrane	384
Other disorders of middle ear and mastoid	385
Vertiginous syndromes and other disorders of vestibular system	386
Otosclerosis	387
Hearing loss	389

Symptoms, signs and ill-defined conditions 780-799

The Ear

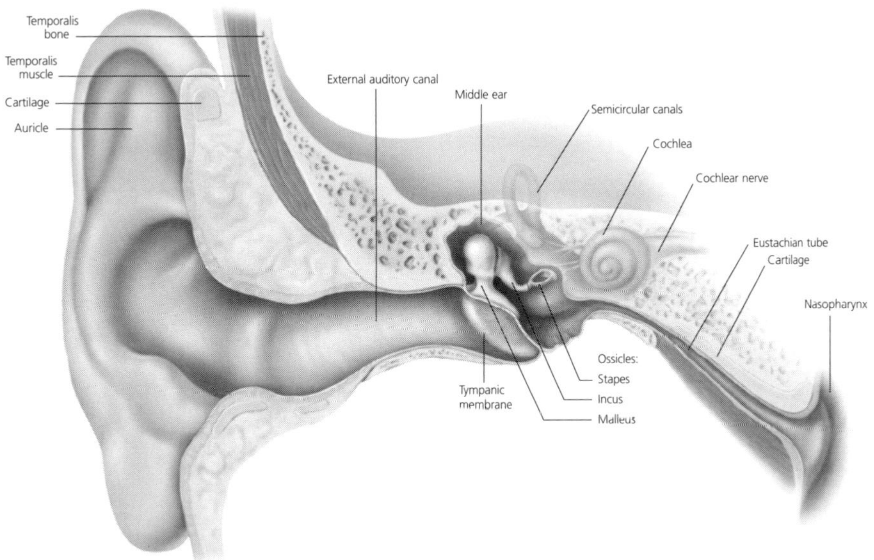

©Scientific Publishing Ltd., Rolling Meadows, IL

ICD-9-CM CODING FUNDAMENTALS

Learning and following the basic steps of coding will increase your chances of better and faster reimbursement from third party payers, as well as establish meaningful profiles for future reimbursement rates. To become a proficient coder, two basic principles must be considered.

First, it is imperative that you use both the Alphabetic Index (Volume 2) and the Tabular List (Volume 1) when locating and assigning codes. Coding only from the Alphabetic Index will cause you to miss any additional information provided only in the Tabular List, such as exclusions, instructions to use additional codes or the need for a fifth-digit. Second, the level of specificity is important in all coding situations. So, a three-digit code that has subdivisions indicates you must use the appropriate subdivision code. Also, any time a fifth-digit subclassification is provided, you must use the fifth-digit code.

NINE STEPS FOR ACCURATE ICD-9-CM CODING

1. Locate the main term within the diagnostic statement.

2. Locate that main term in the Alphabetic Index (Volume 2). Keep in mind that the primary arrangement for main terms is by condition in the Alphabetic Index (Volume 2); main terms can be referred to in outmoded, ill-defined and lay terms as well as proper medical terms; main terms can be expressed in broad or specific terms, as nouns, adjectives or eponyms and can be with or without modifiers. Certain conditions may be listed under more than one main term.

3. Remember to refer to all notes under the main term. Be guided by the instructions in any notes appearing in a box immediately after the main term.

4. Examine any modifiers appearing in parentheses next to the main term. See if any of these modifiers apply to any of the qualifying terms used in the diagnostic statement.

5. Take note of the subterms indented beneath the main term. Subterms differ from main terms in that they provide greater specificity, becoming more specific the further they are indented to the right of the main term in 2-space increments; also, they provide the anatomical sites affected by the disease or injury.

6. Be sure to follow any cross reference instructions. These instructional terms ("see" or "see also") must be followed to locate the correct code.

7. Confirm the code selection in the Tabular List (Volume 1). make certain you have selected the appropriate classification in accordance with the diagnosis.

8. Follow instructional terms in the Tabular List (Volume 1). Watch for exclusion terms, notes and fifth-digit instructions that apply to the code number you are verifying. It is necessary to search not only the selected code number for instructions but also the category, section and chapter in which the code number is collapsible. Many times the instructional information is located one or more pages preceding the actual page you find the code number on.

9. Finally, assign the code number you have determined to be correct.

ITALICIZED ENTRIES: OTHER AND UNSPECIFIED CODES

During the process of designating a code to identify a principal diagnosis it is important to remember that italicized entries or codes in slanted brackets cannot be used. In these instances, it is required that the etiology code be sequenced first and the manifestation code be listed second even if the physician recorded them in the opposite order.

CODING EXERCISE 1

Use both the Alphabetic Index (Volume 2) and the Tabular List (Volume 1) to code the following diagnoses. Identify the main term (MT) and the subterms (ST) for each statement as well.

1. Erythroblastosis fetalis due to RH incompatibility __________
2. Chronic alcoholism, continuous __________
3. Chronic hypertrophy of tonsils __________
4. Acute cholecystitis with bile duct calculus __________
5. Subacute staphylococcal arthritis, knee __________
6. Acute stress reaction __________
7. Bronchial asthma with status asthmaticus __________
8. Bundle branch block __________
9. Food poisoning, bacterial __________
10. Gastric ulcer with perforation __________

Subcategories for diagnoses listed as "Other" and "Unspecified" are referred to as residual subcategories. Remember, the subdivisions are arranged in a hierarchy starting with the more specific and ending with the least specific. In the Tabular List (Volume 1), in most instances, the four-digit subcategory ".8" has been reserved for "Other" specified conditions not classifiable elsewhere and the four-digit subcategory ".9" has been reserved for "Unspecified" conditions. Following is an example demonstrating this principle.

005 Other food poisoning (bacterial)

Excludes: salmonella infections (003.0-003.9)
toxic effect of:
food contaminants (989.7)
noxious foodstuffs (988-0-988.9)

005.0 Staphylococcal food poisoning
Staphylococcal toxemia specified as due to food

005.1 Botulism
Food poisoning due to Clostridium botulinum

005.2 Food poisoning due to Clostridium perfringens
[C. welchii]
Enteritis necroticans

005.3 Food poisoning due to other Clostridia

005.4 Food poisoning due to Vibrio parahaemolyticus

005.8 Other bacterial food poisoning

Excludes: salmonella food poisoning (003.0-003.9)

005.81 Food poisoning due to Vibrio vulnificus

005.89 Other bacterial food poisoning
Food poisoning due to Bacillus cereus

005.9 Food poisoning, unspecified

As you look at Category 005, note that codes 005.0-005.4 indicate that the food poisoning is related to specific types of organisms. Therefore, subcategories 005.0-005.4 are regarded as more specific than subcategory 005.9. Fifth-digit subclassification 005.89, "Other bacterial food poisoning," would include other specific types of bacterial food poisoning not classified elsewhere, as well as bacterial food poisoning, NOS. Whereas, subcategory 005.9, "Food poisoning unspecified," would be used for a diagnostic statement of "Food poisoning NOS" where the causative organism is not mentioned.

The hierarchy from more specific to less specific is not consistently maintained at the fifth-digit level. The level of specificity at the fifth-digit level is usually (not always) indicated by the use of 0 and 9. The digit 9 identifies the entry for "Other specified" while the digit 0 identifies the "Unspecified" entry. Below is an example.

279 Disorders involving the immune mechanism

279.0 Deficiency of humoral immunity

279.00 Hypogammaglobulinemia, unspecified
Agammaglobulinemia NOS

279.01 Selective IgA immunodeficiency

279.02 Selective IgM immunodeficiency

279.03 Other selective immunoglobulin deficiencies
Selective deficiency of IgG

279.04 Congenital hypogammaglobulinemia
Agammaglobulinemia:
Bruton's type
X-linked

279.05 Immunodeficiency with increased IgM
Immunodeficiency with hyper-IgM:
autosomal recessive
X-linked

279.06 Common variable immunodeficiency
Dysgammaglobulinemia (acquired) (congenital) (primary)
Hypogammaglobulinemia:
acquired primary
congenital non-sex-linked
sporadic

279.09 Other

Transient hypogammaglobulinemia of infancy

Notice that the fifth-digit 0 identifies "Unspecified" and the fifth-digit 9 identifies "Other specified."

ACUTE AND CHRONIC CODING

Whenever a particular condition is described as both acute and chronic, code according to the subentries in the Alphabetic Index (Volume 2) for the stated condition. The following directions should be considered.

1. If there are separate subentries listed for acute, subacute and chronic, then use both codes, sequencing the code for the acute condition first.

2. If there are no subentries to identify acute, subacute or chronic, ignore these adjectives when selecting the code for the particular condition.

CODING EXERCISE 2

Code the following diagnostic statements using the steps described above.

1. Allergic rhinitis __________
2. Allergic rhinitis due to dust __________
3. Laryngeal disease __________
4. Laryngeal ulcer __________
5. Polyarthritis __________
6. Polyarthritis of hands, pelvis and knees __________

3. If a certain condition is described as a subacute condition and the index does not provide a subentry designating subacute, then code the condition as if it were acute.

CODING EXERCISE 3

Code the following diagnostic statements relating to Acute and Chronic coding. (Note that the presence of spaces for two codes does not necessarily mean that two codes are required for a particular diagnostic statement).

1. Acute and chronic tonsillitis ________ ________
2. Subacute and chronic endocarditis ________ ________
3. Acute and chronic cholecystitis ________ ________
4. Acute and chronic renal failure ________ ________
5. Subacute and chronic pyelonephritis ________ ________

CODING SUSPECTED CONDITIONS

Whenever the diagnosis is stated as "questionable," "probable," "likely," or "rule out," it is advisable to code documented symptoms or complaints by the patient. The reason for this is that you do not want an insurance carrier to include a disease code in the patient's history if in fact the "suspected" condition is never proven.

Keep in mind that there are no "rule out" codes per se in the ICD-9-CM coding system. If your diagnostic statement is "Rule out Breast Carcinoma" and you use code 174.9 (Malignant Neoplasm of Female Breast, Unspecified), the code definition does not state "rule out." Therefore, the insurance carrier processes the code 174.9 as is, which results in the patient having an insurance history of Malignant Neoplasm, Female Breast, Unspecified.

CODING EXERCISE 4

Code the following diagnostic statements related to "suspected conditions." (Note that the presence of spaces for two codes does not necessarily mean that two codes are required for a particular diagnostic statement).

1. Chest pain, R/O Acute myocardial infarction ________ ________
2. Abdominal discomfort RUQ, possible gall bladder disease ________ ________
3. Fatigue, suspected iron deficiency anemia ________ ________
4. Head trauma, possible cerebral concussion ________ ________
5. Intoxication, probable alcoholism ________ ________
6. SOB, questionable respiratory insufficiency ________ ________
7. Diabetes mellitus ruled out ________ ________

To avoid what could become a problem for you and your patient (including the potential of litigation), you should use codes for signs and symptoms in these cases. For example, use code 611.72 (Lump) or 611.71 (Breast Pain) if these symptoms exist and this is the highest degree of certainty you can code to.

If the patient is asymptomatic but there is a family history of breast cancer then you should consider using a V-code, such as V16.3 (Family history of malignant neoplasm, breast) as your diagnosis code. There are also V-codes to indicate screening for a particular illness or disease. In the above example, code V76.1 (Special screening for malignant neoplasms, breast) could also have been used.

It is important to note that when you use a screening code from the V-code section you should also code signs or symptoms. The reason for doing so is because most health insurance carriers do not provide coverage for routine screening procedures or preventive medicine.

COMBINATION CODES

A combination code is used to fully identify an instance where two diagnoses or a diagnosis with an associated secondary process (manifestation) or complication is included in the description of a single code number. These combination codes are identified by referring to the subterms in the Alphabetic Index (Volume 2) and the inclusion and exclusion terms in the Tabular List (Volume 1).

Examples of commonly used combination codes include 034.0, Streptococcal sore throat and 404, Hypertensive heart and renal disease. Code 034.0 exists because the throat is often infected with Streptococcus and code 404 must be used whenever a patient has both heart and renal disease instead of assigning codes from categories 402 and 403.

Two main terms may be joined together by combination terms listed in the Alphabetic Index (Volume 2) as subterms such as:

associated with	*in*
complicated (by)	*secondary to*
due to	*with*
during	*without*
following	

The listing for the above terms advises the coder to use one or two codes depending on the condition.

MULTIPLE CODING

The concept of multiple coding is encouraged when the use of more than one code number will fully identify a given condition. Thus, use of multiple codes allows all the components of a complex diagnosis to be identified. However, the statement of diagnosis must mention the presence of all the elements for each code number used.

CODING EXERCISE 5

Code the following diagnostic statements related to combination codes.

1. Cholecystitis with bile duct calculus __________
2. Influenza with U.R.I. __________
3. Acute appendicitis with peritoneal abscess __________
4. Skull fracture with subdural hemorrhage __________
5. Salmonella meningitis __________

When is multiple coding mandatory? Only if the instructional term "Code Also" appears in italics under an italicized subdivision in the Tabular List (Volume 1). In this instance, you should interpret mandatory as....requires the use of both codes, and that these codes must be sequenced with the code for the etiology being listed first and the code identifying the manifestation listed as the second code. You will recognize mandatory multiple coding situations by instructional terms used in the Tabular List (Volume 1). The terms to watch for are: "Code Also....," "Use Additional Code...," and "Note:..."

Coding Examples

Cerebral degeneration in childhood with mental retardation

330.9 Unspecified cerebral degeneration in childhood

319 Unspecified mental retardation

Cerebral degeneration in childhood

330.9 Unspecified cerebral degeneration in childhood

If you turn to Category 330 in the Tabular List (Volume 1), you will notice the instructional term cited: "Use additional Code if desired, to identify associated mental retardation." The phrase "...identify associated mental retardation..." should be interpreted as "...identify associated mental retardation, if stated to be present in the diagnostic statement." With this understood, these diagnostic statements would be coded as above.

In the Alphabetic Index (Volume 2), both codes to be used are listed. In this case, the first listed code should be sequenced first with the code in italicized brackets listed second to indicate the additional code. However, the fact that two codes appear after a subterm in the Alphabetic Index does not automatically indicate mandatory multiple coding. It is necessary to verify both code numbers in the Tabular List. If, in the Tabular List, the code number is also in italics as in the Alphabetical Index and, the instructional term "Code Also" appears in italics, then both criteria have been met for mandatory multiple coding.

Coding Example

Diabetic neuropathy

250.60 Diabetes with neurological manifestations

357.2 Polyneuropathy in diabetes

In the Alphabetic Index (Volume 2) you will find Neuropathy listed under Diabetes with the codes 250.6 plus [357.2] in brackets.

It should also be noted at this point, that even though mandatory multiple coding is always indicated by the presence of the instructional term "Code First" in italics beneath the italicized code number and title for the manifestation, this does not always hold true under the code number for the etiology. Multiple coding is not to be used in those instances when a combination code accurately identifies all of the elements within the diagnostic statement.

CODING EXERCISE 6

Code the following diagnostic statements related to multiple coding.

1. Diabetic ulcer, skin ______ ______
2. Viral arthritis ______ ______
3. Malarial fever with hepatitis ______ ______
4. Myocarditis due to tuberculosis ______ ______
5. Endocarditis due to typhoid ______ ______

CODING LATE EFFECTS

You use late effects coding when coding diagnostic statements that identify a residual effect (condition produced) after the acute phase of an illness or injury has ended. The proper coding sequence is the code number identifying the residual (the current condition) to be listed first with the code number identifying the cause (original illness/injury no longer present in its acute phase but which was the cause of the long term residual condition) listed second.

Coding Example

Hemiplegia due to previous cerebral vascular accident

342.90 Hemiplegia, unspecified, affecting unspecified side

438.20 Late effects of cerebrovascular disease, Hemiplegia affecting unspecified side

The residual for this statement is "Hemiplegia" as it is the long term condition that resulted from a previous acute illness. The cause for this statement is "Cerebral vascular accident" as it is the original illness no longer in its acute phase but which did cause the long term residual condition now present. How do you recognize when to use late effects coding and when not to? Often, the diagnostic statement will contain key words to help identify a late effects situation. Key words used in defining late effects include:

late
due to an old injury
due to a previous illness/injury
due to an illness/injury occurring one year or more ago

In cases where these key words (phrases) are not included within the diagnostic statement, an effect is considered to be late if sufficient time has elapsed between the occurrence of the acute illness/injury and the development of the residual effect.

Coding Example

Excessive scar tissue due to third degree burn, right leg

709.2 Scar conditions and fibrosis of skin

906.7 Late effect of burn of other extremities

The previous diagnostic statement does not indicate the time element with any modifying terms as "old" or "previous." The fact that enough time has elapsed for the development of scar tissue indicates that the acute phase of the injury has subsided and the scarring should be coded as a late effect.

CODING EXERCISE 7

Draw a line under the residuals and circle the cause in each of the following diagnostic statements.

1. Contracture right heel tendons due to poliomyelitis
2. Hemiplegia following brain stem injury
3. Malunion of fracture, left humerus
4. Traumatic arthritis due to fracture of left wrist
5. Scoliosis due to radiation

If a diagnostic statement only specifies the cause of the late effect and does not indicate the residual, then use the code number for the cause.

Coding Example

Residuals of tuberculosis

137 Late effects of tuberculosis

The above statement does not identify what the actual residuals are. So, you would use the code for the cause. To find the code for such a statement in the Alphabetic Index (Volume 2), refer to the main term "LATE" and the subterm "EFFECTS OF." The only codes available for causes of late effects are:

137 Late effects of tuberculosis

138 Late effects of acute poliomyelitis

139 Late effects of other infectious and parasitic diseases

268.1 Rickets, late effects

326 Late effects of intracranial abscess or pyogenic infection

438 Late effects of cerebrovascular disease

677 Late effects of complication of pregnancy, childbirth and the puerperium

905 Late effects of musculoskeletal and connective tissue injuries

906 Late effects of injuries to skin and subcutaneous tissues

907 Late effects of injuries to the nervous system

908 Late effects of other and unspecified injuries

909 Late effects of other and unspecified external causes

Be sure to distinguish between a late effect and a historical statement in a diagnosis. Whenever the statement uses the terms "effects of old...," "sequela of...," or "residuals of...," then code as late effects. If the diagnosis is expressed in terms as "history of...," these are coded to personal history of the illness or injury and are coded to the V-Codes (V10 to V19).

CODING EXERCISE 8

Code the following diagnostic statements related to late effects.

1. Mental retardation due to previous viral encephalitis
2. Effects of gunshot wound, right shoulder
3. Brain damage following subdural hematoma 9 months ago
4. Sequela of old crush injury to right hand
5. Malunion of fracture, left humerus

CODING INJURIES

Injuries comprise a major section of ICD-9-CM. Categories 800-959 include fractures, dislocations, sprains and various other types of injuries. Injuries are classified first according to the general type of injury and within each type there is a further breakdown by anatomical site.

In cases where a patient has multiple injuries, the most severe injury is the principal diagnosis. Where multiple sites of injury are specified in the diagnosis, you should interpret the term "with" as indicating involvement of both sites, and interpret the term "and" as indicating involvement of either or both sites. You will also note that fifth digits are commonly used when coding injuries to provide information regarding level of consciousness, specific anatomical sites and severity of injuries.

Some general rules to apply when coding fractures follow. Fractures can either be "open" or "closed." An "open" fracture is when the skin has been broken and there is communication with the bone and the outside of the body. Whereas, with a "closed" fracture the bone does not have contact with the outside of the body.

Note the following descriptions as set forth in the ICD-9-CM at the four-digit subdivision level to help distinguish between an "open" and "closed" fracture.

CLOSED FRACTURES

comminuted	*simple*
linear	*greenstick*
fissured	*depressed*
spiral	*march*
impacted	*fractured nos*
elevated	*slipped epiphysis*

OPEN FRACTURES

compound	*with foreign body*
missile	*infected*
puncture	

Anytime that it is not indicated whether a fracture is "open" or "closed" code it as if it were "closed." Fracture-dislocations are classified as fractures. Pathological fractures are classified to the condition causing the fracture (i.e. osteoporosis) with the use of an additional code to identify the pathological fracture (733.1).

When coding burns, code only the most severe degree of burns when the burns are of the same site but of different degrees. In cases of burns where it is noted that there is an infection, assign the code for the burn and also the code to identify the infection (958.3). The percentage of the body surface involved with burns is specified by using Category 948. This code may be used as a solo code when the site of the burn is unspecified. There is also a fifth-digit subclassification included in Category 948 to identify the percentage of the total body surface involved with third degree burns. Use Category 949 only when neither the site nor the percentage of the body surface involved is specified in the diagnosis.

CODING EXERCISE 9

Code the following diagnostic statements related to injuries.

1. Fracture, right hip __________
2. Comminuted fracture, right ulnar/radius __________
3. Compound fracture, right humerus __________
4. Acute slipped capital femoral epiphysis __________
5. Fracture & dislocation of patella __________
6. Fracture of clavicle with foreign body __________
7. Pathological fracture of lumbar vertebrae due to osteoporosis __________
8. 1st degree and 2nd degree burns of arm __________
9. 3rd degree burn of leg,infected __________
10. 3rd degree burns, 25% of body surface __________
11. 2nd degree burns of back, 18% of body surface __________
12. 1st degree burns __________

POISONING AND ADVERSE EFFECTS OF DRUGS

There are two different sets of code numbers to use to differentiate between poisoning and adverse reactions to the correct substances properly administered. First, you must make the distinction between poisoning and adverse reaction. Poisoning by drugs includes:

ACCIDENTAL

1. Given in error during diagnostic or therapeutic procedures.
2. Given in error by one person to another (for example, mother to child).
3. Taken in error by self.

PURPOSEFUL

1. Suicide attempt.
2. Homicide attempt.

ADVERSE REACTION IN SPITE OF PROPER ADMINISTRATION OF CORRECT SUBSTANCE

1. In therapeutic of diagnostic procedure.
2. Taken by self or given to another as prescribed.
3. Accumulative effect (intoxication due to...).
4. Interaction of prescribed drugs.
5. Synergistic reaction (enhancing the effect of another drug).
6. Allergic reaction.
7. Hypersensitivity.

To code poisoning by drugs, use the Alphabetic Index (Volume 2) which contains the Table of Drugs and Chemicals. This table includes one column to identify the poisoning code (960-989) and four columns of External Cause Codes to classify whether the poisoning was an accident, suicide, assault or undetermined.

The column labeled "Therapeutic Use" is not used for poisonings but in coding adverse reactions to correct substances properly administered. The External Cause Codes are optional but may be used if a facility's coding policy requires their use.

Note that in the Alphabetic Index (Volume 2) that the subterm entry (DRUG) under the main term of poisoning refers the coder to the Table of Drugs and Chemicals for the code assignment. Because the Table of Drugs and Chemicals is so extensive, it is acceptable to code directly from the "Table" without verifying the code obtained in Volume 1.

What if the drug which caused the poisoning is not listed in the Table of Drugs and Chemicals?

1. Refer to Appendix C in Volume 1 (American Hospital Formulary Service) and locate the name of the drug.

2. Note the AHFS category number listed.

3. Turn to the Table of Drugs and Chemicals in the Alphabetic Index (Volume 2).

4. Locate the term "Drug."

5. Refer to the subterm "AHFS LIST."

6. Look through the list until you find the AHFS Category Number determined in step 2 above. The AHFS Category Numbers are listed in numeric order.

7. Assign the code.

HOW DO YOU IDENTIFY POISONING BY DRUGS?

The statement of diagnosis will usually have descriptive terms that would indicate poisoning. Look for terms such as:

Intoxication	*Toxic effect*
Overdose	*Wrong drug given/taken in error*
Poisoning	*Wrong dosage given/taken in error*

Adverse effects of a medicine taken in combination with alcohol or from taking a prescribed drug in combination with a drug the patient took on his/her own initiative (for example antihistamines) are coded as poisonings. If you wish to code a manifestation of the poisoning as well, this code is always listed second, after listing the code identifying the poison first.

CODING EXERCISE 10

Code the following diagnostic statements related to poisoning.

1. Digoxin poisoning __________
2. Morphine overdose __________
3. Adverse reaction to librium with Vodka __________
4. Adverse reaction to Nitroglycerine and over-the-counter antihistamines patient took on his/her own __________
5. Toxic effect of diphtheria vaccine __________
6. Coma due to Valium overdose __________

ADVERSE EFFECTS OF DRUGS

The World Health Organization (WHO) defines adverse drug reaction as any response to a drug "which is noxious and unintended and which occurs at doses used in man for prophylaxis, diagnosis or therapy." Notice that this definition does not include the terms "overdose" or "poisoning."

Why does ICD-9-CM differentiate between poisoning and adverse drug reaction? Tabulation of statistical data indicates how often a drug reaction occurred because of the drug itself versus how often the drug was either not given or taken properly.

Two codes are required when coding adverse drug reactions to the correct substance properly administered. One code is used to identify the manifestation or the nature of the adverse reaction such as urticaria, vertigo, gastritis, etc. This code is assigned from Categories 001-799 in Volume 1.

Refer to the main term identifying the manifestation in the Alphabetic Index (Volume 2). But remember that the Table of Drugs and Chemicals is not used to locate the code for the manifestation, and the code used to identify the manifestation does not identify the drug responsible for the adverse reaction.

A second code is required to identify the drug causing the adverse reaction. In ICD-9-CM, the only codes provided to identify the drug causing an adverse reaction to a substance properly administered are E930 through E949. Anytime a code is selected from the E930-E949 range it can never be sequenced first or stand as a solo code.

LOCATING THE PROPER E CODE

How do you locate the proper E code to identify the drug which was responsible for causing an adverse reaction to a correct substance properly administered? Turn to the Table of Drugs and Chemicals in the Alphabetic Index (Volume 2). Earlier we noted that the column labeled "Therapeutic Use" was not used for coding instances involving poisoning. However, for adverse drug reactions to a correct substance properly administered, the "Therapeutic Use" column is used to find the proper code within the range E930 through E949 to identify the drug.

DRUG INTERACTIONS BETWEEN TWO OR MORE DRUGS

Drug interactions between two or more prescribed drugs are classified as adverse drug reactions to a correct substance properly administered. This holds true regardless of whether the drugs were prescribed by the same physician or different physicians.

Two types of drug interactions should be noted:

1. Synergistic interaction. One drug enhances the action of another drug so that the combined effect is greater than the sum of the effects of each used alone.

2. Antagonistic interaction. One drug represses the action of another drug.

To properly code drug interactions, first code the manifestation. Then code each drug involved in the interaction using the E codes from the column labeled "Therapeutic Use" from the Table of Drugs and Chemicals.

Coding Example

Gastritis due to interaction between Motrin and Procainamide

535.50 Unspecified gastritis and gastroduodenitis
[Manifestation first]

E935.8 Other specified analgesics and antipyretics

E942.0 Cardiac rhythm regulators

When a diagnostic statement does not state specifically the manifestation or nature of the adverse reaction, you should use the code provided to identify an adverse drug reaction of unspecified nature.... 995.2 Unspecified adverse effect of drug, medicinal and biological substance.

Coding Example

Allergic reaction to Motrin, proper dose

995.2 Unspecified adverse effect of drug, medicinal and biological substance

E935.8 Other specified analgesics and antipyretics

Note in the above example that the code indicating the manifestation, although unspecified as to the nature, is listed first followed by the E code to identify the drug. When the drug causing an adverse effect is unknown or unspecified, use code E947.9, Unspecified drug or medicinal substance.

It is very important to remember that codes in the range 960 through 979 are never used in combination with codes in the range E930 through E949 because codes in the range 960-979 identify poisonings and codes in the range E930-E949 identify the external cause of adverse reactions to the correct substance properly administered.

CODING COMPLICATIONS OF MEDICAL AND SURGICAL CARE

A complication is when you have the occurrence of two or more diseases in the same patient. Recent studies have revealed serious deficiencies in properly coding complications for insurance claims processing. Often the complication is never mentioned. Complications are responsible for many of the procedures that are ordered for patients, therefore the complication should be coded and submitted on your insurance claims.

Postoperative complications that affect a specific anatomical site or body system are classified to the appropriate chapter 1 through 16 of the Tabular Index (Volume 1). Postoperative complications affecting more than one anatomical site or body system are classified in the chapter on injury and poisoning (Chapter 17, Categories 996-999). If the Alphabetic Index (Volume 2) does not provide a specific main term and subterm to identify a postoperative complication, classify the complication to categories 996-999.

CODING EXERCISE 11

Code the following diagnostic statements related to adverse effects of drugs. (Note that the presence of spaces for two codes does not necessarily mean that two codes are required for a particular diagnostic statement).

1. Dizziness due to Valium, correct dosage taken ________ ________

2. Blurred vision due to allergic reaction to antihistamines, taken as prescribed ________ ________

3. Aspirin gastritis, taken as recommended ________ ________

4. Electrolyte imbalance due to interaction between Lithium carbonate and diuretic ________ ________

5. Drug allergy ________ ________

6. Percodan hypersensitivity ________ ________

Coding Examples

Postcholecystectomy syndrome

576.0 Postcholecystectomy syndrome

The Alphabetic Index (Volume 2) specifically classifies the postoperative condition to one of the categories from 001 through

799. See main term "complication," subterms "surgical procedure" and "postcholecystectomy syndrome."

Postoperative wound infection

998.5 Postoperative infection

The Alphabetic Index (Volume 2) has a main term "infection" and subterms "wound, postoperative" for this condition. Note that this code appears in Chapter 17 within categories 996-999.

Postoperative atelectasis

997.3 Complications affecting specified body systems, not elsewhere classified; Respiratory complications

Refer to the main term "atelectasis" in the Alphabetic Index (Volume 2). Note there is no subterm for postoperative beneath this main term. Therefore, you must presume this complication is classified to one of the categories in the range 969-999. You may also code 518.0 to identify the nature of the respiratory complication for statistical purposes; however, the code for the complication must be listed first.

COMPLICATIONS FROM MECHANICAL DEVICES

Subcategories in the range 996.0 through 996.5 are used to identify mechanical complications of devices. Mechanical complications are the result of a malfunction on the part of the internal prosthetic implant or device. What indicates a mechanical complication? Breakdown or obstruction, displacement, leakage, perforation or protrusion of the devices are all forms of mechanical complications.

Coding Examples

Displacement of cardiac pacemaker electrode

996.01 Mechanical complication of cardiac device, implant and graft due to cardiac pacemaker (electrode)

Protrusion of nail into acetabulum

996.4 Mechanical complications of internal orthopedic device, implant, and graft.

Other complications of devices, such as infection or hemorrhage, are due to an abnormal reaction of the body to an otherwise properly functioning device. All complications involving infection are coded to category 996.7, Other complications of internal (biological) (synthetic) prosthetic device, implant and graft.

Coding Examples

Infected arteriovenous shunt

996.6 Infection and inflammatory reaction due to internal prosthetic device, implant, and graft

Anterior chamber hemorrhage due to displaced prosthetic lens

996.7 Other complications of internal (biological) (synthetic) prosthetic device, implant, and graft

SPECIAL NOTES REGARDING CARDIAC COMPLICATIONS

In the case of cardiac complications, ICD-9-CM defines the "immediate postoperative period" as "the period between surgery and the time of discharge from the hospital." This definition is the basis of whether to code cardiac complications under subcategory 997.1, Complications affecting specified body systems, not elsewhere classified, cardiac complications, or under subcategory 429.4, Ill-defined descriptions and complications of heart disease, functional disturbances following cardiac surgery.

You will code with subcategory 997.1 for a cardiac complication that occurs anytime between surgery and hospital discharge from any type of procedure performed. Subcategory 429.4 is used to code long-term cardiac complications resulting from cardiac surgery.

It is important to distinguish between complications and aftercare. Aftercare is usually an encounter for something planned in advance (example, removal of Kirshner wire). Aftercare is classified using codes in the range of V51-V58. An encounter for a complication occurs from unforeseen circumstances, such as wound infection, resulting in complication of the patient's condition.

SPECIAL CODING SITUATIONS

As you become an experienced coder you will encounter situations where the standard rules do not seem to apply, or which require a special understanding in order to code properly. These situations include coding of circulatory diseases, diabetes, mental disorders, infectious diseases, manifestations, neoplasms, and pregnancy and childbirth. This chapter addresses these specific special coding situations.

CODING CIRCULATORY DISEASES

Because of the variety of terms and phrases used by physicians to identify diseases of the circulatory system, you will often experience difficulty in coding. To accurately code disorders of the circulatory system, it is imperative that the coder carefully read all inclusion, exclusion and "use additional code" notations contained in the Tabular List (Volume 1).

Fifth digit subclassifications are also frequently used to code combination disorders or to provide further specificity in this section. Even those in specialties other than cardiology will frequently find themselves coding circulatory system diagnoses due to the prevalence of circulatory disorders in this country.

Chapter 7 of the Tabular List (Volume 1), titled Diseases of Circulatory System, contains the following major sections:

1.	Acute Rheumatic Fever	390-392
2.	Chronic Rheumatic Heart Disease	393-398
3.	Hypertensive Disease	401-405
4.	Ischemic Heart Disease	410-414
5.	Diseases of Pulmonary Circulation	415-417

6. Other Forms of Heart Disease 420-429

7. Cerebrovascular Disease 430-438

8. Diseases of Arteries, Arterioles, and Capillaries 440-448

9. Diseases of Veins and Lymphatics, and Other Diseases of Circulatory System 451-459

DISEASES OF MITRAL AND AORTIC VALVES

Certain diseases of the mitral valve of unspecified etiology are presumed to be of rheumatic origin and others are not. None of the disorders of the aortic valve of unspecified etiology are presumed to be of rheumatic origin. When you have disorders involving both the mitral and aortic valves of unspecified etiology, then they are presumed to be of rheumatic origin.

Coding Examples

Mitral Valve Insufficiency

424.0 Other diseases of endocardium
Mitral valve disorders

Refer to the main term "insufficiency" in the Alphabetic Index (Volume 2). Note the subterm "mitral (valve)."

Mitral Valve Stenosis

394.0 Diseases of mitral valve
Mitral stenosis

Refer to the main term "stenosis" and the sub-term "mitral (valve)" in the Alphabetic Index (Volume 2).

Aortic Valve Insufficiency

424.1 Other diseases of endocardium
Aortic valve disorders

Aortic valve stenosis

424.1 Other diseases of endocardium
Aortic valve disorders

Look up the main term "stenosis" and the subterm "aortic" in the Alphabetic Index (Volume 2). Remember that aortic valve disorders of unspecified etiology are not considered rheumatic in nature or origin.

Insufficiency of mitral and aortic valves

396.3 Diseases of mitral and aortic valves
Mitral valve insufficiency and
aortic valve insufficiency

Under the main term "insufficiency" in the Alphabetic Index (Volume 2) you will find the subterm "aortic." Further review will locate "with," "mitral valve disease," "insufficiency, incompetence or regurgitation" which directs you to code 396.3.

ISCHEMIC HEART DISEASE

In ischemic heart disease, the manifestations are due to a lack of blood flow to the heart rather than to the anatomical lesion of the coronary arteries. The most common cause of coronary heart disease is coronary atherosclerosis. However, ischemic heart disease can be due to non-coronary disease, such as aortic valvular stenosis, as well. There are many synonyms used to indicate ischemic heart disease such as: coronary artery heart disease, ASHD, and coronary ischemia. Categories in the range 410-414, Ischemic Heart Disease, includes that with mention of hypertension. Use an additional code to identify the presence of hypertension.

Coding Examples

Angina pectoris

413.9 Other and unspecified angina pectoris

As no mention of hypertension is made in the diagnostic statement, a single code is all that is required.

Angina pectoris with essential hypertension

413.9 Other and unspecified angina pectoris

401.9 Essential hypertension, Unspecified

In this example, the mention of hypertension in the diagnostic statement requires the use of a second code.

MYOCARDIAL INFARCTION

A myocardial infarction is classified as acute if it is either specified as "acute" in the diagnostic statement or with a stated duration of eight weeks or less. When a myocardial infarction is specified as "chronic" or with symptoms after eight weeks from the date of the onset, it should be coded to subcategory 414.8, Other specified forms of chronic ischemic heart disease. If a myocardial infarction is specified as old or healed or has been diagnosed by special investigation (EKG) but is currently not presenting any symptoms, code using category 412, Old myocardial infarction.

Coding Examples

Myocardial infarction three weeks ago

410.9 Acute myocardial infarction, Unspecified site

Chronic myocardial infarction with angina

414.8 Other specified forms of chronic ischemic heart disease

413.9 Other and unspecified angina pectoris

Myocardial infarction diagnoses by EKG, symptomatic

412 Old myocardial infarction

ARTERIOSCLEROTIC CARDIOVASCULAR DISEASE (ASCVD)

Arteriosclerotic cardiovascular disease (ASCVD) is classified to subcategory 429.2, Cardiovascular disease, Unspecified. You should use an additional code to identify the presence of arteriosclerosis when coding ASCVD. For example, the diagnostic statement "generalized arterio-sclerotic cardiovascular disease" should be coded using 429.2 followed by 440.9.

Other forms of heart disease, categories 420-429, are used for multiple coding purposes to fully identify a stated diagnosis. The exception to this rule is if the Alphabetic Index (Volume 2) or Tabular List (Volume 1) specifically instructs you otherwise.

Coding Examples

Arteriosclerotic heart disease with acute pulmonary edema

428.1 Left heart failure

414.0 Coronary atherosclerosis

Note that the code for ASHD (414.0) is listed second as a possible underlying cause of the acute situation.

Arteriosclerotic heart disease with congestive heart failure

428.0 Congestive heart failure

414.0 Coronary atherosclerosis

CEREBROVASCULAR DISEASE

When coding cerebrovascular disease (codes 430-438), you should code the component parts of the diagnostic statement identifying the cerebrovascular disease, unless specifically instructed to do otherwise in the Alphabetic Index (Volume 2) or Tabular List (Volume 1).

Coding Examples

Cerebrovascular arteriosclerosis with subarachnoid hemorrhage

430 Subarachnoid hemorrhage

437.0 Cerebral atherosclerosis

Cerebrovascular accident secondary to thrombosis

434.0 Cerebral thrombosis

In this example, you use only one code because of the instructions in the Alphabetic Index (Volume 2). When you look up the main term "accident" with subterm "cerebrovascular," you are instructed to "see also" disease, cerebrovascular, acute (436). When you locate the main term "disease" and subterms "cerebrovascular," "acute," and "thrombotic" you are further instructed to "see" thrombosis, brain. This is where you finally locate the single code for this diagnosis... 434.0.

Whenever there are conditions resulting from the acute cerebrovascular disease, code them if they are stated to be residual(s). If the resulting condition is stated to be transient, do not code them.

Coding Examples

Cerebrovascular accident with residual aphasia

436 Acute, but ill-defined, cerebrovascular disease

784.3 Aphasia

Cerebrovascular accident with transient hemiparesis

436 Acute, but ill-defined, cerebrovascular disease

HYPERTENSIVE DISEASE

As demonstrated earlier with ischemic heart disease, conditions that are classified to cerebrovascular disease (codes 430-438) include that with mention of hypertension, but you must identify the hypertension with another code (401-405) and list it second.

Hypertensive disease is classified to the categories 401-405. The Table of Hypertension is located in the Alphabetic Index (Volume 2) under the main term "Hypertension." This Table contains subterms to identify types of hypertension and complications as well as three columns labeled "malignant," "benign," and "unspecified" as to whether malignant or benign.

cardiovascular disease (arteriosclerotic) (sclerotic)	402.00	402.10	402.90
with			
heart failure (congestive)	402.01	402.11	402.91
renal involvement (conditions classifiable to 403) (*see also* Hypertension, cardiorenal)	404.00	404.10	404.90
cardiovascular renal (disease) (sclerosis) (*see also* Hypertension cardiorenal)	404.00	404.10	404.90
cerebrovascular disease NEC	437.2	437.2	437.2
complicating pregnancy, childbirth, or the puerperium . . .	642.2	642.0	642.9
with			
albuminuria (and edema) (mild)	—	—	642.4
severe	—	—	642.5
edema (mild)	—	—	642.4
severe	—	—	642.5
heart disease	642.2	642.2	642.2
and renal disease	642.2	642.2	642.2
renal disease	642.2	642.2	642.2
and heart disease	642.2	642.2	642.2
chronic	642.2	642.0	642.0
with pre-eclampsia or eclampsia	642.7	642.7	642.7
fetus or newborn	760.0	760.0	760.0
essential	—	642.0	642.0
with pre-eclampsia or eclampsia	—	642.7	642.7
fetus or newborn	760.0	760.0	760.0

Hypertension is frequently the cause of various forms of heart and vascular disease. However, the mention of hypertension with some heart conditions should not be interpreted as a combination resulting in hypertensive heart disease. The combination is only to be made if there is a cause-and-effect relationship between hypertension and a heart condition classified to subcategories 425.8, 428.0-428.9, 429.0-429.3 and 429.8-429.9.

First you need to be able to make a distinction between conditions specified as "due to" or "with" hypertension. Keep in mind that the phrase "due to hypertension" and the word "hypertensive" are to be considered synonymous.

Coding Examples

Hypertensive heart disease

402.90 Hypertensive heart disease, Unspecified, Without congestive heart failure

Heart disease due to hypertension

402.90 Hypertensive heart disease, Unspecified, Without congestive heart failure

Each of the above diagnostic statements indicate clearly a cause-and-effect relationship between hypertension and the condition by specifying that the condition is "due to." Therefore, both statements are coded using 402.90.

If the phrase "with hypertension" is stated or, the diagnostic statement mentions the conditions separately, then you code the conditions separately.

Coding Example

Myocarditis with hypertension

429.0 Myocarditis, Unspecified

401.9 Essential hypertension, Unspecified

As a cause-and-effect relationship is not indicated in the diagnostic statement, the conditions are coded separately.

HIGH BLOOD PRESSURE VERSUS ELEVATED BLOOD PRESSURE

With the ICD-9-CM coding system there is a differentiation made between high blood pressure (hypertension) and elevated blood pressure without a diagnosis of hypertension. If the diagnostic statement indicates elevated blood pressure without the diagnosis of hypertension, it is coded to subcategory 796.2, Elevated blood pressure reading without diagnosis of hypertension. If the diagnostic statement indicates high blood pressure or hypertension, it is coded to Category 401, Essential hypertension.

CODING EXERCISE 12

Code the following diagnostic statements related to circulatory diseases. (Note that the presence of spaces for two codes does not necessarily mean that two codes are required for a particular diagnostic statement).

1. Mitral valve regurgitation ________ ________
2. Aortic valve stenosis, rheumatic ________ ________
3. Arteriosclerotic heart disease with hypertension ________ ________
4. Acute coronary insufficiency ________ ________
5. Atherosclerotic coronary artery disease; angina pectoris ________ ________
6. Acute myocardial infarction; ASHD ________ ________

CODING EXERCISE 12 continued...

7. Old anterior wall myo- cardial infarction __________ __________

8. Angina pectoris secondary to chronic myocardial infarction __________ __________

9. Atherosclerotic cardio- vascular degeneration __________ __________

10. Arteriosclerotic disease with gangrene of right lower extremity __________ __________

11. Vertebral artery insuf- ficiency with transient vertigo __________ __________

12. Acute CVA with residual hemiparesis __________ __________

13. Benign essential hyper- tension __________ __________

14. Hypertensive renal failure __________ __________

15. Hypertension due to renal artery stenosis __________ __________

16. Congestive heart failure with hypertension __________ __________

17. Left heart failure with benign hypertension __________ __________

18. Dizziness; elevated blood pressure __________ __________

DIABETES MELLITUS CODING (250)

In 1980, the American Diabetic Association reclassified the types of diabetes mellitus to signify whether or not the patient is dependent on insulin for survival of life. In 1994, additional classifications were added. Note the revisions (bracketed portions) of the statements below for the fifth-digit subclassification.

0 type II [non-insulin dependent type][NIDDM type][adult-onset type] or unspecified type, not stated as uncontrolled

1 type I [insulin dependent type][IDDM][juvenile type], not stated as uncontrolled

2 type II [non-insulin dependent type][NIDDM][adult-onset type] or unspecified type, uncontrolled

3 type I [insulin dependent type][IDDM][juvenile type], uncontrolled

Fifth digit 0 is for use with type II, adult onset diabetic patients, even if the patient requires insulin

Fifth digit 2 is for use with type II, adult onset diabetic patients, even if the patient requires insulin

Do not assume a patient has insulin-dependent diabetes simply because the patient is receiving insulin, as some non-dependent diabetics may require temporary use when they encounter stressful situations such as surgery or physical or mental illness.

Any time diabetes is described as "brittle" or "uncontrolled" you should interpret it as diabetes mellitus complicated and assign code 250.9 with the appropriate fifth digit, 0, 1, 2 or 3. However, if there is also a specific complication present, then assign the code identifying that specific complication, for example, diabetes mellitus, brittle, with ketoacidosis — 250.12 or 250.13.

CODING EXERCISE 13

Code the following diagnostic statements related to diabetes mellitus. (Note that the presence of spaces for two codes does not necessarily mean that two codes are required for a particular diagnostic statement).

1. Diabetic cataract ________ ________
2. Diabetic gangrene ________ ________
3. Diabetes mellitus, juvenile, brittle with neuropathy ________ ________
4. Diabetes mellitus, hyperosmotic, nonketotic coma, insulin dependent ________ ________
5. Diabetes mellitus, uncontrolled ________ ________

CODING MENTAL DISORDERS

You should be aware of the existence of the glossary of mental disorders in Appendix B of the Tabular List (Volume 1). This glossary is not used for coding purposes but rather as a guide to provide a common frame of reference for statistical comparisons. It is simply an alphabetized listing of mental disorders with definitions.

The coder should choose code assignments based on the terminology used by the physician or psychiatrist and not by the coder's impression of the content of the categories and subcategories. The chapter on mental disorders has many fifth digit subclassifications to watch for when selecting your code.

Adjustment reaction or disorder: Mild or transient disorders lasting longer than acute stress reactions which occur in individuals of any age without any apparent pre-existing mental disorder. Such disorders are often relatively circumscribed or situation-specific, are generally reversible, and usually last only a few months. They are usually closely related in time and content to stresses such as bereavement, migration, or other experiences. Reactions to major stress that last longer than a few days are also included. In children such disorders are associated with no significant distortion of development.[1]

conduct disturbance: Mild or transient disorders in which the main disturbance predominantly involves a disturbance of conduct (e.g., an adolescent grief reaction resulting in aggressive or antisocial disorder).[1]

depressive reaction: States of depression, not specifiable as manic-depressive, psychotic, or neurotic.[1]

brief: Generally transient, in which the depressive symptoms are usually closely related in time and content to some stressful event.[1]

prolonged: Generally long-lasting, usually developing in association with prolonged exposure to a stressful situation.[1]

emotional disturbance: An adjustment disorder in which the main symptoms are emotional in type (e.g., anxiety, fear, worry) but not specifically depressive.[1]

mixed conduct and emotional disturbance: An adjustment reaction in which both emotional disturbance and disturbance of conduct are prominent features.[1]

Affective psychoses: Mental disorders, usually recurrent, in which there is a severe disturbance of mood (mostly compounded of depression and anxiety but also manifested as elation, and excitement) which is accompanied by one or more of the following: delusions, perplexity, disturbed attitude to self, disorder of perception and behavior; these are all in keeping with the individual's prevailing mood (as are hallucinations when they occur). There is a strong tendency to suicide. For practical reasons,

Sample of the Glossary of Mental Disorders

INFECTIOUS AND PARASITIC DISEASES

There are two categories for identifying the organism causing diseases classified elsewhere.

041 Bacterial infection in conditions classified elsewhere and of unspecified site

079 Viral and chlamydial infection in conditions classified elsewhere and of unspecified site

These codes may be used as either additional codes, or as solo codes depending on the diagnostic statement.

Coding Examples

Acute UTI due to Escherichia coli

599.0 Urinary tract infection, site not specified

041.4 Escherichia coli

Staphylococcus infection

041.11 Staphylococcus aureus

Bacterial infection

041.9 Bacterial infection, unspecified

The basic coding principles regarding combination codes (one code accurately identifies the components of the condition) applies throughout the chapter on Infectious and Parasitic Diseases.

In the Alphabetic Index (Volume 2), a subterm that identifies an infectious organism takes precedence in code assignment over a subterm at the same indentation level that identifies a site or other descriptive term.

Coding Example

Chronic syphilitic cystitis

095.8 Other specified forms of late symptomatic syphilis

Using the Alphabetic Index (Volume 2) to look up the main term "cystitis (bacillary)," you will note the subterms "Chronic 595.2" and "Syphilitic 095.8" at the same indentation level under the main term. Therefore, code 095.8 is assigned to this diagnostic statement, as the organism has precedence over other descriptive terms or anatomical sites.

CODING EXERCISE 14

Code the following diagnostic statements related to infectious and parasitic diseases. (Note that the presence of spaces for two codes does not necessarily mean that two codes are required for a particular diagnostic statement).

1. Moniliasis of vulva _________ _________
2. Pneumonia due to Staphylococcus aureus _________ _________
3. Periurethral abscess due to Streptococcus _________ _________
4. Staphylococcal food poisoning _________ _________
5. Mental retardation secondary to previous viral infection _________ _________
6. Empyema due to Streptococcal infection _________ _________

MANIFESTATIONS

Manifestations are characteristic signs or symptoms of an illness. Signs and symptoms that point rather definitely to a given diagnosis are assigned to the appropriate chapter of ICD-9-CM, for example, hematuria is assigned to the Genitourinary System chapter. However, Chapter 16, Symptoms, Signs, and Ill-Defined Conditions (780-799), includes ill-defined conditions and symptoms that may suggest two or more diseases or, may point to two or more systems of the body, and are used in cases lacking the necessary study to make a final diagnosis.

Conditions allocated to Chapter 16 include:

1. Cases for which no more specific diagnosis can be made even after all facts bearing on the case have been investigated; for example code 784.0, Headache.

2. Signs or symptoms existing at the time of initial encounter that proved to be transient and whose cause could not be determined; for example code 780.2, Syncope and collapse.

3. Provisional diagnoses in a patient who failed to return for further investigation or care; for example code 782.4, Jaundice, unspecified, not of newborn.

4. Cases referred elsewhere for investigation or treatment before the diagnosis was made; for example code 782.5, Cyanosis.

5. Cases in which a more precise diagnosis was not available for any other reason; for example code 780.7, Malaise and fatigue.

6. Certain symptoms which represent important problems in medical care and which it might be desired to classify in addition to a known cause; for example, code 780.01, Coma.

In the latter case, if the cause of a symptom or sign is stated in the diagnosis, assign the code identifying the cause. An additional code may be assigned to further identify this symptom or sign if a need to further identify the symptom or sign has been identified. In such cases, the code identifying the cause will ordinarily be listed as the principal diagnosis.

CODING OF NEOPLASMS

The coding of neoplasms requires a good understanding of medical terminology. All neoplasms are classified to Chapter 2 of the Tabular List (Volume 1) under Neoplasms (140-239), which contains the following broad groups:

140-195 Malignant neoplasms, stated or presumed to be primary, of specified sites, except of lymphatic and hematopoietic tissue.

196-198	Malignant neoplasms, stated or presumed to be secondary, of specified sites.
199	Malignant neoplasms, without specification of site.
200-208	Malignant neoplasms, stated or presumed to be primary, of lymphatic and hematopoietic tissue.
210-229	Benign neoplasms.
230-234	Carcinoma in situ.
235-238	Neoplasms of uncertain behavior.
239	Neoplasms of unspecified nature.

TABLE OF NEOPLASMS

The Table of Neoplasms appears in the Alphabetic Index (Volume 2) under the main term "Neoplasms." This table gives the code numbers for neoplasms of anatomical site. For each anatomical site there are six possible code numbers according to whether the neoplasm in questions is either:

- Malignant:
  - Primary
  - Secondary
  - Ca in situ
- Benign
- Of uncertain behavior
- Of unspecified nature

	Malignant					
	Primary	Secondary	Ca in situ	Benign	Uncertain Behavior	Unspecified
esophagogastric junction	151.0	197.8	230.2	211.1	235.2	239.0
esophagus	150.9	197.8	230.1	211.0	235.5	239.0
abdominal	150.2	197.8	230.1	211.0	235.5	239.0
cervical	150.0	197.8	230.1	211.0	235.5	239.0
contiguous sites	150.8	—	—	—	—	—
distal (third)	150.5	197.8	230.1	211.0	235.5	239.0
lower (third)	150.5	197.8	230.1	211.0	235.5	239.0
middle (third)	150.4	197.8	230.1	211.0	235.5	239.0
proximal (third)	150.3	197.8	230.1	211.0	235.5	239.0
specified part NEC	150.8	197.8	230.1	211.0	235.5	239.0
thoracic	150.1	197.8	230.1	211.0	235.5	239.0
upper (third)	150.3	197.8	230.1	211.0	235.5	239.0
ethmoid (sinus)	160.3	197.3	231.8	212.0	235.9	239.1
bone or labyrinth	170.0	198.5	—	213.0	238.0	239.2
Eustachian tube	160.1	197.3	231.8	212.0	235.9	239.1
exocervix	180.1	198.82	233.1	219.0	236.0	239.5
external						
meatus (ear)	173.2	198.2	232.2	216.2	238.2	239.2

The Table of Neoplasms appears in the Alphabetic Index (Volume 2)

DEFINITIONS OF SITE AND BEHAVIORS OF NEOPLASMS

PRIMARY Identifies the stated or presumed site of origin.

SECONDARY Identifies site(s) to which the primary site has spread (direct extension) or metastasized by lymphatic spread, invading local blood vessels, or by implantation as tumor cells shed into body cavities.

BENIGN Tumor does not invade adjacent structures or spread to distant sites but may displace or exert pressure on adjacent structures.

IN-SITU Tumor cells that are undergoing malignant changes but are still confined to the point of origin without invasion of surrounding normal tissue (non-infiltrating, non-invasive or pre-invasive carcinoma).

OF UNCERTAIN BEHAVIOR	The pathologist is not able to determine whether the tumor is benign or malignant because some features of each are present.
UNSPECIFIED NATURE	Neither the behavior nor the histological type of tumors are specified in the diagnostic statement. This type of diagnosis may be encountered when the patient has been treated elsewhere and comes in terminally ill without accompanying information, is referred elsewhere for work-up, or no work-up is performed because of advanced age or poor condition of the patient.

STEPS TO CODING NEOPLASMS

1. ICD-9-CM disregards classification of neoplasms by histological type (according to tissue origin) with the exception of lymphatic and hematopoietic neoplasms, malignant melanoma of skin, lipoma, and a few common tumors of bone, uterus, ovary, etc. All other tumors are classified by system, organ or site. The existence of these exceptions makes it neccssary to first consult the Alphabetic Index (Volume 2) to determine whether a specific code has been assigned to a specified histological type. For example, Malignant melanoma of skin of scalp is coded 172.4 although the code specified in the "Malignant: Primary Column" of the Neoplasm Table for skin of scalp is 173.4.

2. The General Alphabetical Index (Volume 2) also provides guidance to the appropriate column for neoplasms which are not assigned a specific code by histological type. For example, if you look up Lipomyoma, specified site in the Alphabetic Index (Volume 2), you will find "See Neoplasm, connective tissue, benign."

   The guidance in the Alphabetic Index (Volume 2) can be overridden if a descriptor is present. For example, Malignant adenoma of colon is coded as 153.9 and not as 211.3 because the adjective "malignant" overrides the entry "adenoma - See also Neoplasm, benign."

3. The Neoplasm Table may be consulted directly if a specific neoplasm diagnosis indicates which column of the table is appropriate but does not delineate a specific type of tumor.

4. Sites marked with an asterisk (*), such as buttock NEC* or calf*, should be classified to malignant neoplasm of skin of these sites if the variety of neoplasm is a squamous cell carcinoma or an epidermoid carcinoma and to benign neoplasm of skin of these sites if the variety of neoplasm is a papilloma (of any type).

5. Primary malignant neoplasms are classified to the site of origin of the neoplasm. In some cases, it may not be possible to identify the site of origin, such as malignant neoplasms originating from contiguous sites.

   Neoplasms with overlapping site boundaries are classified to the fourth-digit subcategory .8 "other." For example, code 151.8 "Malignant neoplasm of contiguous or overlapping sites of stomach whose point of origin cannot be determined."

6. Neoplasms which demonstrate functional activity require an additional code to identify the functional activity.

   Coding Example

   Cushing's syndrome due to malignant pheochromocytoma

   194.0 Malignant neoplasm of adrenal gland

   255.0 Disorders of adrenal glands; Cushing's syndrome

   Code sequencing depends on the circumstances of the encounter.

7. Two codes in the malignant neoplasm section represent departures from the usual principles of classification in that the fourth-digit subdivisions in each case are not mutually exclusive. These codes are 150 "Malignant neoplasms of the esophagus" and 201 "Hodgkin's disease." The dual axis is provided to account for differing

terminology, for there is no uniform international agreement on the use of these terms.

Coding Example

Malignant neoplasm of the esophagus

150.0 Cervical esophagus

150.1 Thoracic esophagus

150.2 Abdominal esophagus

or using alternate coding

150.3 Upper third of esophagus

150.4 Middle third of esophagus

150.5 Lower third of esophagus

8. When the treatment is directed at the primary site of the malignancy, designate the primary site as the principal diagnosis, except when the encounter or hospital admission is solely for radiotherapy session(s), code V58.0 or, for chemotherapy sessions, V58.1.

9. When surgical intervention for removal of a primary site or secondary site malignancy is followed by adjunct chemotherapy or radiotherapy, code the malignancy using codes in the 140-198 series, or, where appropriate, in the 200-203 series as long as chemotherapy or radiotherapy is being actively administered. If the admission is for chemotherapy or radiotherapy, the malignancy code is listed second.

10. When the primary malignancy has been previously excised or eradicated from its site and there is no adjunct treatment directed to that site and, there is no evidence of any remaining malignancy at the primary site, use the appropriate code from the V10 series to indicate the site of the primary malignancy. Any mention of extension, invasion or metastasis to a nearby structure or organ, or to a distant

site is coded as a secondary malignant neoplasm to that site and may be the principal diagnosis in the absence of the primary site.

11. If the patient has no secondary malignancy and if the reason for admission or for the visit is follow-up of the malignancy, two codes are used and sequenced as follows:

Coding Example

Follow-up of breast cancer treated with chemotherapy. No evidence of recurrence.

V67.2 Follow-up examination following chemotherapy

V10.3 Personal history of carcinoma of breast

12. Malignancies of hematopoietic and lymphatic tissue are always coded to the 200.0-208.9 series unless specified as "in remission." In remission is coded as V10.60-V10.79.

13. If the primary malignant neoplasm previously excised or eradicated has recurred, code it as primary malignancy of the stated site unless the Alphabetic Index (Volume 2) directs you to do otherwise.

Coding Examples

Recurrence of prostate carcinoma

185 Malignant neoplasm of the prostate

Recurrence of breast carcinoma in mastectomy site

198.2 Secondary malignant neoplasm of other specified sites, skin of breast

Make sure to code any mention of secondary site(s).

14. Terminology referring to metastatic cancer is often ambiguous, so when there is doubt as to the meaning intended, the following rules should be used:

    A. Cancer "metastatic from" a site should be interpreted as primary of that site.

    B. Cancer described as "metastatic to" a site should be interpreted as secondary of that site.

    Coding Examples

    Carcinoma in axillary lymph nodes and lungs metastatic from breast

    174.9 Malignant neoplasm of female breast, unspecified

    196.3 Secondary and unspecified malignant neoplasm of lymph nodes of axilla and upper limb

    197.0 Secondary malignant neoplasm of lung

    Adenocarcinoma of colon with extension to peritoneum

    153.9 Malignant neoplasm of colon, unspecified

    197.6 Secondary malignant neoplasm of retroperitoneum and peritoneum

15. Diagnostic statements when only one site is identified as metastatic:

    A. Code to the category for "primary of unspecified site" for the morphological type concerned UNLESS the code thus obtained is either 199.0 or 199.1.

B. If the code obtained in the above step is 199.0 or 199.1, then code the site qualified as "metastatic" as for a primary malignant neoplasm of the stated site EXCEPT for the sites listed below, which should always be coded as secondary neoplasm of the state site:

Bone	Mediastinum
Brain	Meninges
Diaphragm	Peritoneum
Heart	Pleura
Liver	Retroperitoneum
Lymph nodes	Spinal cord

Sites classifiable to 195

C. Also assign the appropriate code for primary or secondary malignant neoplasm of specified or unspecified site, depending on the diagnostic statement you are coding.

Coding Examples

Metastatic renal cell carcinoma of lung

189.0 Malignant neoplasm of kidney, except pelvis

197.0 Secondary malignant neoplasm of lung

Metastatic carcinoma of lung

162.9 Malignant neoplasm of bronchus and lung, unspecified

199.1 Malignant neoplasm without specification of site, other

This code is assigned to identify "secondary neoplasm of unspecified site" per the instructions in step C above.

Metastatic carcinoma of brain

198.3 Secondary malignant neoplasm of other specified sites, brain and spinal cord

199.1 Malignant neoplasm without specification of site, other

In this case, the brain is one of the sites listed in Step B as an exception. So, for this diagnostic statement, the code assignment is for secondary neoplasm of the brain and primary malignant neoplasm of unspecified site.

16. When two or more sites are stated in the diagnostic statement and all are qualified to be "metastatic," you should code as for "primary site unknown" and code the stated sites as secondary neoplasms of those sites.

Coding Example

Metastatic melanoma of lung and liver

172.9 Malignant melanoma of skin, site unspecified

197.0 Secondary malignant neoplasm of lung

197.7 Secondary malignant neoplasm of liver, specified as secondary

17. When there is no site specified in the diagnostic statement, but the morphological type is qualified as "metastatic," code as for "primary site unknown." Then, assign the code for secondary neoplasms of unspecified site.

Coding Example

Metastatic apocrine adenocarcinoma

173.9 Other malignant neoplasms of skin, site unspecified

199.1 Malignant neoplasm without specification of site, other

18. When two or more sites are stated in the diagnosis and only some are qualified as "metastatic" while others are not, code as for "primary site unknown." However, you should interpret the following sites as secondary neoplasms:

Bone	Meninges
Brain	Peritoneum
Diaphragm	Pleura
Heart	Retroperitoneum
Liver	Spinal Cord

Sites classifiable to category 195

Coding Example

Carcinoma of lung, metastatic, and brain

198.3 Secondary malignant neoplasm of brain and spinal cord

197.0 Secondary malignant neoplasm of lung

199.1 Malignant neoplasm without specification of site, other

PREGNANCY, CHILDBIRTH, AND THE PUERPERIUM

Chapter 11 of the Tabular List (Volume 1) uses fifth-digit subclassifications extensively. In general, the fifth digit is not given in the Alphabetic Index (Volume 2), so each code must be verified in the Tabular List (Volume 1).

The codes for Ectopic and Molar Pregnancy, 630-633, do not require the fifth digit. Note also that for the codes 634-638, there is a "common" set of fourth-digit subcategory codes to include complications. Be aware of the use of section marks with categories 634-637 to indicate the need for a fifth digit. All other codes, 640-676, require the use of a fifth digit with the single exception of code 650, Normal delivery.

Coding Example

Pregnancy, 3 months gestation complicated by benign essential hypertension

642.03 Benign essential hypertension complicating pregnancy, childbirth, and the puerperium, antepartum condition or complication

Categories 647 and 648 are used for conditions that are usually classified elsewhere, but which have been classified here because they are complications of pregnancy. The interaction of certain conditions with the pregnant state complicates the pregnancy and/or aggravates the non-obstetrical condition (i.e., diabetes mellitus, drug dependence, thyroid dysfunction) and are the main reasons for the obstetrical care provided.

Coding Examples

Rubella in woman, 7 months gestation

647.53 Infectious and parasitic conditions in the mother classifiable elsewhere, but complicating pregnancy, childbirth, or the puerperium, rubella, antepartum condition or complication

Pregnancy with diabetes mellitus

648.03 Other current conditions in the mother classifiable elsewhere, but complicating pregnancy, childbirth, or the puerperium, diabetes mellitus, antepartum condition or complication

If greater detail is needed for the complication, use an additional code to identify the complication more completely.

Coding Example

Pregnancy with pernicious anemia

648.23 Other current conditions in the mother classifiable elsewhere, but complicating pregnancy, childbirth, or the puerperium, anemia, antepartum condition or complication

281.0 Pernicious anemia

USING V CODES

V codes are used to identify encounters with the health care setting for reasons other than an illness or injury, for example, immunization. V codes are also used to identify encounters of persons who are injured or ill and whose injury or illness is influenced by some circumstance or problem classified to the V codes, for example, a person with a functioning pacemaker who requires emergency gastrointestinal surgery. V codes fall into one of three categories; problems, services or factual.

1. Problem V codes identify a circumstance or problem that could affect a patient's overall health status but is not itself a current illness or injury. In other words, you may note that a patient has a drug allergy to sulfonamides by using code V14.2 - Personal History of Allergy to Sulfonamides. Although this allergy is not considered an illness or a problem in a healthy person, it may affect how the physician will actually care for the patient. You would only use a problem V code when the problem has a potential effect on the patient's current diagnosis and the physician's treatment plan for management of the illness or injury.

2. Service V codes describe circumstances other than an illness or injury which prompt the patient's visit. This type of visit often occurs when the patient has a chronic disease but is not acutely ill. An example would be a patient with a known neoplasm that has sought care to receive chemotherapy. In this instance, you would assign the V code V58.1 - Maintenance Chemotherapy as the primary code on your

claim and list the code to identify the known neoplasm second.

3. Factual V codes are used to describe certain facts that do not fall into the "problem" or "service" categories. For example, coding the type of birth using code V30.1 - Single Liveborn, born before admission to hospital.

V codes can be used as a solo code, a principal code or as a secondary code. It is important to use V codes properly. If a complication is present, the complication should be coded to categories 001-799 instead of to a V code.

Coding Example

Colostomy status with colostomy malfunction

569.60 Colostomy and enterostomy complication, unspecified

[Code V44.3 - Artificial opening status, colostomy] would not be used in this case because of the complication.

Key words found in diagnostic statements which may result in selection of a V code include:

Admission for
Aftercare
Attention to
Care (of)
Carrier
Checking/checkup
Contact
Contraception
Counseling
Dialysis
Donor
Examination
Fitting of
Follow up
Health or healthy
History (of)
Maintenance
Maladjustment
Observation
Problem (with)
Prophylactic
Replacement (by)(of)
Screening
Status
Supervision (of)
Test
Transplant
Vaccination

CODING EXERCISE 15

Code the following diagnostic statements related to V codes. (Note that the presence of spaces for two codes does not necessarily mean that two codes are required for a particular diagnostic statement).

1. Routine pap smear, cervix including gynecologic exam _________ _________
2. Chemotherapy in office for treatment of malignant neoplasm of lung _________ _________
3. Removal of screw from healed fracture, arm _________ _________
4. Replace cystostomy tube _________ _________
5. Patient fell from ladder at work. No injury on exam. _________ _________

USING E CODES

E codes permit the classification of environmental events, circumstances and conditions as the cause of injury, poisoning and other adverse effects. The use of E codes together with the code identifying the injury or condition provides additional information of particular concern to industrial medicine, insurance carriers, national safety programs and public health agencies.

The E codes may be assigned with any of the codes in the main classification 001-999 to identify the external cause of an injury or condition. E codes are *never* used as solo codes or as principal diagnostic codes.

When using E codes, search the Alphabetic Index (Volume 2) for the main term identifying the cause such as "accident," "fire," "shooting," "fall," or "collision." To find the E code for an adverse reaction to surgical or medical treatment, use the main term "reaction."

Coding Example

Burns to right arm, occurred while burning trash

943.00 Burn of upper limb, except wrist and hand, unspecified degree
E897 Accident caused by controlled fire not in building or structure

E-codes are important for providing the details of an accident to an insurance carrier to enable them to issue faster and more accurate reimbursement. Most insurance carriers want to be sure they reimburse only for services covered under their policy and not for services covered under Worker's Compensation, Automobile or Homeowner's insurance. A clear understanding of the circumstances will eliminate questions from the insurance carrier which cause delays in reimbursements.

Coding Example

Fractured ribs due to fall from ladder at home

807.00 Fracture of ribs, closed, unspecified

E881.0 Fall from ladder

E849.0 Place of occurrence, home

Using the above E codes to provide important information regarding the circumstances of the injury to the insurance carrier eliminates any doubt about the insurer's responsibility for coverage.

When using E codes, always list the E codes as secondary or supplemental to the code(s) describing the injury.

APPENDIX A

ANSWERS TO CODING EXERCISES

CODING EXERCISE 1

1.	Erythroblastosis (MT) fetalis due to RH (ST) incompatibility	773.0
2.	Chronic (ST) alcoholism (MT), continuous	303.91
3.	Chronic hypertrophy (MT) of Tonsils (ST)	474.11
4.	Acute cholecystitis (MT) with bile duct calculus (ST)	574.30
5.	Subacute staphylococcal (ST) arthritis (MT), knee	711.06
6.	Acute stress (MT/ST) reaction (MT/ST)	308.9
7.	Bronchial (ST) asthma (MT) with status asthmaticus	493.91
8.	Bundle (ST) branch block (MT)	426.50
9.	Food (MT) poisoning (MT), bacterial (ST)	005.9
10.	Gastric (ST) ulcer (MT) with perforation	531.50

MT = main term, ST = subterm

CODING EXERCISE 2

1.	Allergic rhinitis	477.9
2.	Allergic rhinitis due to dust	477.8
3.	Laryngeal disease	478.70
4.	Laryngeal ulcer	478.79

5. Polyarthritis	711.90 or 716.59
6. Polyarthritis of hands, pelvis and knees	711.98 or 716.58

CODING EXERCISE 3

1. Acute and chronic tonsillitis	463 & 474.00
2. Subacute and chronic endocarditis	421.9 & 424.90
3. Acute and chronic cholecystitis	575.12
4. Acute and chronic renal failure	584.9 & 585
5. Subacute and chronic pyelonephritis	590.10 & 590.00

CODING EXERCISE 4

1. Chest pain, R/0 Myocardial Infarction	786.50 & V81.0 or V71.7
2. Abdominal discomfort RUQ, possible gallbladder disease	789.01 & V71.8 or V82.8
3. Fatigue, suspected iron deficiency anemia	780.7 & V78.0
4. Head trauma, possible cerebral concussion	854.00 & V80.0
5. Intoxication, probable alcoholism	305.00 & V79.1
6. SOB, questionable respiratory insufficiency	786.09 & V81.4
7. Diabetes mellitus ruled out	V77.1

CODING EXERCISE 5

1. Cholecystitis with bile duct calculus — 574.40
2. Influenza with URI — 487.1
3. Acute appendicitis with peritoneal abscess — 540.1
4. Skull fracture with subdural hemorrhage — 803.20
5. Salmonella meningitis — 003.21

CODING EXERCISE 6

1. Diabetic ulcer, skin — 250.80 & 707.9
2. Viral arthritis — 079.99 & 711.50
3. Malarial fever with hepatitis — 084.9 & 573.2
4. Myocarditis due to tuberculosis — 017.9 & 422.0
5. Endocarditis due to typhoid — 002.0 & 421.1

CODING EXERCISE 7

1. Contracture right heel tendons due to (poliomyelitis)
2. Hemiplegia following (brain stem injury)
3. Malunion of (fracture), left humerus
4. Traumatic arthritis due to (fracture) of left wrist
5. Scoliosis due to (radiation)

CODING EXERCISE 8

1.	Mental retardation due to previous viral encephalitis	319 & 139.0
2.	Effects of gunshot wound, right shoulder	906.1
3.	Brain damage following subdural hematoma, 9 months ago	348.9 & 907.0
4.	Sequela of old crush injury to right hand	906.4
5.	Malunion of fracture, left humerus	733.81 & 905.2

CODING EXERCISE 9

1.	Fracture, right hip	820.8
2.	Comminuted fracture, right humerus	812.20
3.	Compound fracture, right humerus	812.30
4.	Acute slipped capital femoral epiphysis	732.2
5.	Fracture and dislocation of patella	822.0
6.	Fracture of clavicle with foreign body	810.10
7.	Pathological fracture of lumbar vertebrae due to osteoporosis	733.13
8.	First-degree and second-degree burns of arm	943.20
9.	Third-degree burn of leg, infected	945.30 & 958.3
10.	Third-degree burns, 25% body surface	948.22
11.	Second-degree burns of back, 18% of body surface	942.24 & 948.1

12. First-degree burns	949.1

CODING EXERCISE 10

1. Digoxin poisoning	972.1
2. Morphine overdose	965.09
3. Adverse reaction to Librium and Vodka	969.4
4. Adverse reaction to Nitroglycerine and over-the-counter antihistamines patient took on his own	972.4
5. Toxic effect of diphtheria vaccine	978.5
6. Coma due to Valium overdose	969.4 & 780.01

CODING EXERCISE 11

1. Dizziness due to Valium, correct dosage taken	780.4 & E939.4
2. Blurred vision due to allergic reaction to antihistamines, taken as prescribed	368.8 & E933.0
3. Aspirin gastritis, medication taken as recommended	535.50 & E935.3
4. Electrolyte imbalance due to interaction between Lithium carbonate and diuretic	276.9 & E939.8 & E944.4
5. Drug allergy	995.2 & E947.9
6. Percodan hypersensitivity	995.2 & E935.2

CODING EXERCISE 12

1. Mitral valve regurgitation	424.0
2. Aortic valve stenosis, rheumatic	395.0

3.	Arteriosclerotic heart disease with hypertension	401.9 & 414.00
4.	Acute coronary insufficiency	411.89
5.	Atherosclerotic coronary artery disease; angina syndrome	414.00 & 413.9
6.	Acute myocardial infarction, arteriosclerotic heart disease	410.90 & 414.00
7.	Old anterior wall myocardial infarction	412
8.	Angina pectoris secondary to chronic myocardial infarction	413.9 & 412
9.	Atherosclerotic cardiovascular degeneration	429.2 & 414.00
10.	Arteriosclerotic disease with gangrene of right lower extremity	785.4 & 414.00
11.	Vertebral artery insufficiency with transient vertigo	435.1
12.	Acute CVA with residual hemiparesis	436 & 342.90
13.	Benign essential hypertension	401.1
14.	Hypertensive renal failure	403.91
15.	Hypertension due to renal artery stenosis	405.91
16.	Congestive heart failure with hypertension	428.0 & 401.9
17.	Left heart failure with benign hypertension	428.1 & 401.1
18.	Dizziness; elevated blood pressure	780.4 & 796.2

CODING EXERCISE 13

1. Diabetic cataract — 250.50 & 366.41
2. Diabetic gangrene — 250.70 & 785.4
3. Diabetes mellitus, juvenile, brittle with neuropathy — 250.63 & 357.2
4. Diabetes mellitus, hyperosmotic, nonketotic coma, insulin dependent — 250.21
5. Diabetes mellitus, uncontrolled — 250.92

CODING EXERCISE 14

1. Moniliasis of vulva — 112.1
2. Pneumonia due to Staphylococcus aureus — 482.41
3. Periurethral abscess due to Streptococcus aureus — 597.0 & 041.00
4. Staphylococcal food poisoning — 005.0
5. Mental retardation secondary to previous viral infection — 319 & 079.99
6. Empyema due to Streptococcal infection — 510.9 & 041.00

CODING EXERCISE 15

1. Routine pap smear, cervix including gynecological exam — V72.3
2. Chemotherapy in office for treatment of malignant neoplasm of lung — V58.1 & 162.9
3. Removal of screw from healed fracture, arm — V54.0

4. Replace cystostomy tube V55.5

5. Patient fell from ladder at work. No injury on exam. V71.3

APPENDIX B

LIST OF THREE-DIGIT CATEGORIES

1. INFECTIOUS AND PARASITIC DISEASES

Intestinal infectious diseases	001-009
Tuberculosis	010-018
Zoonotic bacterial diseases	020-027
Other bacterial diseases	030-041
Human immunodeficiency virus (HIV)	042
Poliomyelitis and other non-arthropod-borne viral diseases of central nervous system	045-049
Viral diseases accompanied by exanthem	050-057
Arthropod-borne viral diseases	060-066
Other diseases due to viruses and Chlamydiae	070-079
Rickettsioses and other arthropod-borne diseases	080-088
Syphilis and other venereal diseases	090-099
Other spirochetal diseases	100-104
Mycoses	110-118
Helminthiasis	120-129
Other infectious and parasitic diseases	130-136

Late effects of infectious and parasitic diseases	137-139

2. NEOPLASMS

Malignant neoplasm of lip, oral cavity, and pharynx	140-149
Malignant neoplasm of digestive organs and peritoneum	150-159
Malignant neoplasm of respiratory and and intrathoracic organs	160-165
Malignant neoplasm of bone, connective tissue, skin, and breast	170-176
Malignant neoplasm of genitourinary organs	179-189
Malignant neoplasm of other and unspecified sites	190-199
Malignant neoplasm lymphatic and hematopoietic tissue	200-208
Benign neoplasms	210-229
Carcinoma in situ	230-234
Neoplasms of uncertain behavior	235-238
Neoplasms of unspecified behavior	239

3. ENDOCRINE, NUTRITIONAL AND METABOLIC DISEASES, AND IMMUNITY DISORDERS

Disorders of thyroid gland	240-246
Diseases of other endocrine glands	250-259

Nutritional deficiencies	260-269
Other metabolic disorders and immunity disorders	270-279

4. DISEASES OF BLOOD AND BLOOD-FORMING ORGANS

Anemias	280-285
Other diseases of blood and blood-forming organs	286-289

5. MENTAL DISORDERS

Organic psychotic conditions	290-294
Other psychoses	295-299
Neurotic disorders, personality disorders and other nonpsychotic mental disorders	300-316
Mental retardation	317-319

6. DISEASES OF THE NERVOUS SYSTEM AND SENSE ORGANS

Inflammatory diseases of the central nervous system	320-326
Hereditary and degenerative diseases of the central nervous system	330-337
Other disorders of the central nervous system	340-349
Disorders of the peripheral nervous system	350-359
Disorders of the eye and adnexa	360-379
Diseases of the ear and mastoid process	380-389

7. DISEASES OF THE CIRCULATORY SYSTEM

Acute rheumatic fever	390-392
Chronic rheumatic heart disease	393-398
Hypertensive disease	401-405
Ischemic heart disease	410-414
Diseases of pulmonary circulation	415-417
Other forms of heart disease	420-429
Cerebrovascular disease	430-438
Diseases of arteries, arterioles, and capillaries	440-448
Diseases of veins and lymphatics, and other diseases of circulatory system	451-459

8. DISEASES OF THE RESPIRATORY SYSTEM

Acute respiratory infections	460-466
Other diseases of upper respiratory tract	470-478
Pneumonia and influenza	480-487
Chronic obstructive pulmonary disease and allied conditions	490-496
Pneumoconioses and other lung diseases due to external agents	500-508
Other diseases of respiratory system	510-519

9. DISEASES OF THE DIGESTIVE SYSTEM

Diseases of oral cavity, salivary glands, and jaws	520-529
Diseases of esophagus, stomach, and and duodenum	530-537
Appendicitis	540-543
Hernia of abdominal cavity	550-553
Noninfective enteritis and colitis	555-558
Other diseases of intestines and peritoneum	560-569
Other diseases of digestive system	570-579

10. DISEASES OF THE GENITOURINARY SYSTEM

Nephritis, nephrotic syndrome, and nephrosis	580-589
Other diseases of urinary system	590-599
Diseases of male genital organs	600-608
Disorders of breast	610-611
Inflammatory disease of female pelvic organs	614-616
Other disorders of female genital tract	617-629

11. COMPLICATIONS OF PREGNANCY, CHILDBIRTH, AND THE PUERPERIUM

Ectopic and molar pregnancy	630-633
Other pregnancy with abortive outcome	634-639
Complications mainly related to pregnancy	640-648
Normal delivery, and other indications for care in pregnancy, labor and delivery	650-659
Complications occurring mainly in the course of labor and delivery	660-669
Complications of the puerperium	670-677

12. DISEASES OF THE SKIN AND SUBCUTANEOUS TISSUE

Infections of skin and subcutaneous tissue	680-686
Other inflammatory conditions of skin and subcutaneous tissue	690-698
Other diseases of skin and subcutaneous tissue	700-709

13. DISEASES OF THE MUSCULOSKELETAL SYSTEM AND CONNECTIVE TISSUE

Arthropathies and related disorders	710-719
Dorsopathies	720-724
Rheumatism, excluding the back	725-729
Osteopathies, chondropathies, and acquired musculoskeletal deformities	730-739

14. CONGENITAL ANOMALIES

Congenital anomalies	740-759

15. CERTAIN CONDITIONS ORIGINATING IN THE PERINATAL PERIOD

Maternal causes of perinatal morbidity and mortality	760-763
Other conditions originating in the perinatal period	764-779

16. SYMPTOMS, SIGNS, AND ILL-DEFINED CONDITIONS

Symptoms	780-789
Nonspecific abnormal findings	790-796
Ill-defined and unknown causes of morbidity and mortality	797-799

17. INJURY AND POISONING

Fracture of skull	800-804
Fracture of neck and trunk	805-809
Fracture of upper limb	810-819
Fracture of lower limb	820-829
Dislocation	830-839
Sprains and strains of joints and adjacent muscles	840-848
Intracranial injury, excluding those with skull fracture	850-854

Internal injury of thorax, abdomen, and pelvis	860-869
Open wound of head, neck, and trunk	870-879
Open wound of upper limb	880-887
Open wound of lower limb	890-897
Injury to blood vessels	900-904
Late effects of injuries, poisonings, toxic effects, and other external causes	905-909
Superficial injury	910-919
Contusion with intact skin surface	920-924
Crushing injury	925-929
Effects of foreign body entering through orifice	930-939
Burns	940-949
Injury to nerves and spinal cord	950-957
Certain traumatic complications and unspecified injuries	958-959
Poisoning by drugs, medicinal and biological substances	960-979
Toxic effects of substances chiefly nonmedicinal as to source	980-989
Other and unspecified effects of external causes	990-995

Complications of surgical and medical care, not elsewhere classified	996-999

18. SUPPLEMENTARY CLASSIFICATION OF FACTORS INFLUENCING HEALTH STATUS AND CONTACT WITH HEALTH SERVICES (V CODES)

Persons with potential health hazards related to communicable diseases	V01-V06
Persons with need for isolation, other potential health hazards and prophylactic measures	V07-V09
Persons with potential health hazards related to personal and family history	V10-V19
Persons encountering health services in circumstances related to reproduction and development	V20-V29
Liveborn infants according to type of birth	V30-V39
Persons with a condition influencing their health status	V40-V49
Persons encountering health services for specific procedures and aftercare	V50-V59
Persons encountering health services in other circumstances	V60-V69
Persons without reported diagnosis encountered during examination and investigation of individuals and populations	V70-V82

APPENDIX C

CODES REQUIRING 4TH OR 5TH DIGIT

1. INFECTIOUS AND PARASITIC DISEASES

Categories and Subcategories	Fifth Digits
003.2	0,1,2,3,4,9
005.8	1,9
008.0	0,1,2,3,4,9
008.4 and 008.6	1,2,3,4,5,6,7,9
010 - 018	0,1,2,3,4,5,6
032.8	1,2,3,4,5,9
036.4	0,1,2,3
036.8	1,2,9
038.1	0,1,9
038.4	0,1,2,3,4,9
040.8	1,9
041.0	0,1,2,3,4,5,9
041.1	0,1,9
041.8	1,2,3,4,5,6,9
045	0,1,2,3
053.1	0,1,2,3,9
053.2	0,1,2,9
053.7	1,9
054.1	0,1,2,3,9
054.4	0,1,2,3,4,9
054.7	1,2,3,9
055.7	1,9

Categories and Subcategories	Fifth Digits
056.0	0,1,9
056.7	1,9
070.2 and 070.3	0,1,2,3
070.4 and 070.5	1,2,3,4,9
072.7	1,2,9
074.2	0,1,2,3
077.9	8,9
078.1	0,1,9
078.8	1,2,8,9
079.5	0,1,2,3,9
079.8	1,8,9
079.9	8,9
082.4	0,1,9
088.8	1,2,9
090.4	0,1,2,9
091.5	0,1,2
091.6	1,2,9
091.8	1,2,9
093.2	0,1,2,3,4
093.8	1,2,9
094.8	1,2,3,4,5,6,7,9
098.1	0,1,2,3,4,5,6,7,9
098.3	0,1,2,3,4,5,6,7,9
098.4	0,1,2,3,9
098.8	1,2,3,4,5,6,9
099.4	0,1,9
099.5	0,1,2,3,4,5,6,9

Categories and Subcategories	Fifth Digits
100.8	1,9
112.8	1,2,3,4,5,9
115	0,1,2,3,4,5,9
131.0	0,1,2,3,9

2. NEOPLASMS

198.8	1,2,9
200 - 202	0,1,2,3,4,5,6,7,8
203 - 208	0,1
223.8	1,9
228.0	0,1,2,3,4,9
236.9	0,1,9
237.7	0,1,2

3. ENDOCRINE, NUTRITIONAL, METABOLIC & IMMUNITY

242	0,1
250	0,1,2,3
274.1	0,1,9
274.8	1,2,9
275.4	0,1,2,9
277.0	0,1
278.0	0,1
279.0	0,1,2,3,4,5,6,9
279.1	0,1,2,3,9

4. BLOOD AND BLOOD-FORMING ORGANS

282.6	0,1,2,3,9

Categories and Subcategories	Fifth Digits
283.1	0,1,9
285.2	1,2,9
289.5	0,1,9

5. MENTAL DISORDERS

290.1	0,1,2,3
290.2	0,1
290.4	0,1,2,3
291.8	1,9
292.1	1,2
292.8	1,2,3,4,9
293.8	1,2,3,4,9
294.1	0,1
295	0,1,2,3,4,5
296.0 - 296.6	0,1,2,3,4,5,6
296.8	0,1,2,9
296.9	0,9
299	0,1
300.0	0,1,2,9
300.1	0,1,2,3,4,5,6,9
300.2	0,1,2,3,9

Categories and Subcategories	Fifth Digits
300.8	1,2,9
301.1	0,1,2,3
301.2	0,1,2
301.5	0,1,9
301.8	1,2,3,4,9
302.5	0,1,2,3
302.7	0,1,2,3,4,5,6,9
302.8	1,2,3,4,5,9
303 - 304	0,1,2,3
305.0, 305.2-305.9	0,1,2,3
306.5	0,1,2,3,9
307.2	0,1,2,3
307.4	0,1,2,3,4,5,6,7,8,9
307.5	0,1,2,3,4,9
307.8	0,1,9
309.2	1,2,3,4,8,9
309.8	1,2,3,9
312.0 - 312.2	0,1,2,3
312.3	0,1,2,3,4,5,9
312.8	1,2,9
313.2	1,2,3
313.8	1,2,3,9
314.0	0,1
315.0	0,1,2,9
315.3	1,2,9

Categories and Subcategories	Fifth Digits
6. NERVOUS SYSTEM	
320.8	1,2,9
331.8	1,9
333.8	1,2,3,4,9
333.9	0,1,2,3,9
335.1	0,1,9
335.2	0,1,2,3,4,9
337.2	0,1,2,9
342	0,1,2
344.0	0,1,2,3,4,9
344.3 and 344.4	0,1,2
344.6	0,1
344.8	1,9
345.0 - 345.1	0,1
345.4 - 345.9	0,1
346	0,1
349.8	1,2,9
355.7	1,9
360.0	0,1,2,3,4
360.1	1,2,3,4,9
360.2	0,1,3,4,9
360.3 & 360.4	0,1,2,3,4
360.5 & 360.6	0,1,2,3,4,5,9
360.8	1,9
361.0	0,1,2,3,4,5,6,7
361.1	0,1,2,3,4,9
361.3	0,1,2,3

Categories and Subcategories	Fifth Digits
361.8	1,9
362.0	1,2
362.1	0,1,2,3,4,5,6,7,8
362.2	1,9
362.3	0,1,2,3,4,5,6,7
362.4	0,1,2,3
362.5	0,1,2,3,4,5,6,7
362.6	0,1,2,3,4,5,6
362.7	0,1,2,3,4,5,6,7
362.8	1,2,3,4,5,9
363.0	0,1,3,4,5,6,7,8
363.1	0,1,2,3,4,5
363.2	0,1,2
363.3	0,1,2,3,4,5
363.4	0,1,2,3
363.5	0,1,2,3,4,5,6,7
363.6	1,2,3
363.7	0,1,2
364.0	0,1,2,3,4,5
364.1	0,1
364.2	1,2,3,4
364.4	1,2
364.5	1,2,3,4,5,6,7,9
364.6	0,1,2,3,4
364.7	0,1,2,3,4,5,6,7
365.0	0,1,2,3,4

Categories and Subcategories	Fifth Digits
365.1	0,1,2,3,4,5
365.2	0,1,2,3,4
365.3	1,2
365.4	1,2,3,4
365.5	1,2,9
365.6	0,1,2,3,4,5
365.8	1,2,9
366.0	0,1,2,3,4,9
366.1	0,1,2,3,4,5,6,7,8,9
366.2	0,1,2,3
366.3	0,1,2,3,4
366.4	1,2,3,4,5,6
366.5	0,1,2,3
367.2	0,1,2
367.3	1,2
367.5	1,2,3
367.8	1,9
368.0	0,1,2,3
368.1	0,1,2,3,4,5,6
368.3	0,1,2,3,4
368.4	0,1,2,3,4,5,6,7
368.5	1,2,3,4,5,9
368.6	0,1,2,3,9
369.0 and 369.1	0,1,2,3,4,5,6,7,8
369.2	0,1,2,3,4,5
369.6	0,1,2,3,4,5,6,7,8,9
369.7	0,1,2,3,4,5,6

Categories and Subcategories	Fifth Digits
370.0	0,1,2,3,4,5,6,7
370.2	0,1,2,3,4
370.3	1,2,3,4,5
370.4	0,4,9
370.5	0,2,4,5,9
370.6	0,1,2,3,4
371.0	0,1,2,3,4,5
371.1	0,1,2,3,4,5,6
371.2	0,1,2,3,4
371.3	0,1,2,3
371.4	0,1,2,3,4,5,6,8,9
371.5	0,1,2,3,4,5,6,7,8
371.6	0,1,2
371.7	0,1,2,3
371.8	1,2,9
372.0 and 372.1	0,1,2,3,4,5
372.2	0,1,2
372.3	0,1,3,9
372.4	0,1,2,3,4,5
372.5	0,1,2,3,4,5,6
372.6	1,2,3,4
372.7	1,2,3,4,5
372.8	1,9
373.0	0,1,2
373.1	1,2,3
373.3	1,2,3,4
374.0	0,1,2,3,4,5

Categories and Subcategories	Fifth Digits
374.1	0,1,2,3,4
374.2	0,1,2,3
374.3	0,1,2,3,4
374.4	1,3,4,5,6
374.5	0,1,2,3,4,5,6
374.8	1,2,3,4,5,6,7,9
375.0	0,1,2,3
375.1	1,2,3,4,5,6
375.2	0,1,2
375.3	0,1,2,3
375.4	1,2,3
375.5	1,2,3,4,5,6,7
375.6 and 375.8	1,9
376.0	0,1,2,3,4
376.1	0,1,2,3
376.2	1,2
376.3	0,1,2,3,4,5,6
376.4	0,1,2,3,4,5,6,7
376.5	0,1,2
376.8	1,2,9
377.0	0,1,2,3,4
377.1	0,1,2,3,4,5,6
377.2	1,2,3,4
377.3	0,1,2,3,4,9
377.4	1,2,9
377.5	1,2,3,4

Categories and Subcategories	Fifth Digits
377.6	1,2,3
377.7	1,2,3,5
378.0	0,1,2,3,4,5,6,7,8
378.1	0,1,2,3,4,5,6,7,8
378.2	0,1,2,3,4
378.3	0,1,2,3,4,5
378.4	0,1,2,3,4,5
378.5	0,1,2,3,4,5,6
378.6	0,1,2,3
378.7	1,2,3
378.8	1,2,3,4,5,6,7
379.0	0,1,2,3,4,5,6,7,9
379.1	1,2,3,4,5,6,9
379.2	1,2,3,4,5,6,9
379.3	1,2,3,4,9
379.4	0,1,2,3,5,6,9
379.5	0,1,2,3,4,5,6,7,8,9
379.9	0,1,2,3,9
380.0	0,1,2
380.1	0,1,2,3,4,5,6
380.2	1,2,3
380.3	0,1,2,9
380.5	0,1,2,3
380.8	1,9
381.0	0,1,2,3,4,5,6
381.1	0,9

Categories and Subcategories	Fifth Digits
381.2	0,9
381.5	0,1,2
381.6	0,1,2,3
381.8	1,9
382.0	0,1,2
383.0	0,1,2
383.2	0,1,2
383.3	0,1,2,3
383.8	1,9
384.0	0,1,9
384.2	0,1,2,3,4,5
384.8	1,2
385.0	0,1,2,3,9
385.1	0,1,2,3,9
385.2	1,2,3,4
385.3	0,1,2,3,5
385.8	2,3,9
386.0	0,1,2,3,4
386.1	0,1,2,9
386.3	0,1,2,3,4,5
386.4	0,1,2,3,8
386.5	0,1,2,3,4,5,6,8
388.0	0,1,2
388.1	0,1,2
388.3	0,1,2
388.4	0,1,2,3,4

Categories and Subcategories	Fifth Digits
388.6	0,1,9
388.7	0,1,2
389.0	0,1,2,3,4,8
389.1	0,1,2,4,8

7. CIRCULATORY SYSTEM

Categories and Subcategories	Fifth Digits
398.9	0,1,9
402	0,1
403	0,1
404	0,1,2,3
405	1,9
410	0,1,2
411.8	1,9
414.0	0,1,2,3,4,5
414.1	0,1,9
415.1	1,9
420.9	0,1,9
422.9	0,1,2,3,9
424.9	0,1,9
426.1	0,1,2,3
426.5	0,1,2,3,4
426.8	1,9
427.3	1,2
427.4	1,2
427.6	0,1,9
427.8	1,9
429.7	1,9

Categories and Subcategories	Fifth Digits
429.8	1,2,9
433 and 434	0,1
438.1	0,1,2,9
438.2	0,1,2
438.3	0,1,2
438.4	0,1,2
438.5	0,1,2,3
438.8	1,2,9
440.2	0,1,2,3,4,9
440.3	0,1,2
441.0	0,1,2,3
442.8	1,2,3,4,9
443.8	1,9
444.2	1,2
444.8	1,9
446.2	0,1,9
451.1	1,9
451.8	1,2,3,4,9
456.2	0,1
459.8	1,9

8. RESPIRATORY SYSTEM

464.1	0,1
464.2	0,1
464.3	0,1
466.1	1,9
474.0	0,1,2

Categories and Subcategories	Fifth Digits
474.1	0,1,2
478.2	0,1,2,4,5,6,9
478.3	0,1,2,3,4
478.7	0,1,4,5,9
482.3	0,1,2,9
482.4	0,1,9
482.8	1,2,3,4,9
491.2	0,1
493	0,1,2
518.8	1,2,3,4,9
519.0	0,1,2,9

9. DIGESTIVE SYSTEM

Categories and Subcategories	Fifth Digits
524.0	0,1,2,3,4,5,6,9
524.1	0,1,2,9
524.6	0,1,2,3,9
524.7	0,1,2,3,4,9
526.8	1,9
530.1	0,1,9
530.8	1,2,3,4,9
531 - 535	0,1
536.4	0,1,2,9
537.8	1,2,3,9
550	0,1,2,3
551.0	0,1,2,3
551.2	0,1,9

Categories and Subcategories	Fifth Digits
552.0	0,1,2,3
552.2	0,1,9
553.0	0,1,2,3
553.2	0,1,9
560.3	0,1,9
560.8	1,9
562.0	0,1,2,3
562.1	0,1,2,3
564.8	1,9
568.8	1,2,9
569.4	1,2,9
569.6	0,1,2,9
569.8	1,2,3,4,5,9
571.4	0,1,9
574	0,1
575.1	0,1,2

10. THE GENITOURINARY SYSTEM

Categories and Subcategories	Fifth Digits
580.8	1,9
581.8	1,9
582.8	1,9
583.8	1,9
590.0	0,1
590.1	0,1
590.8	0,1
593.7	0,1,2,3

Categories and Subcategories	Fifth Digits
593.8	1,2,9
595.8	1,2,9
596.5	1,2,3,4,5,9
597.8	0,1,9
598.0	0,1
599.8	1,2,3,4,9
604.9	0,1,9
607.8	1,2,3,4,9
608.8	1,3,4,5,6,9
611.7	1,2,9
616.1	0,1
616.5	0,1

11. PREGNANCY, CHILDBIRTH & PUERPERIUM

634 - 637	0,1,2
640 - 641	0,1,3
642	0,1,2,3,4
643	0,1,3
644.0 and 644.1	0,3
644.2	0,1
645.1 and 645.2	0,1,3
646.0	0,1,3
646.1 and 646.2	0,1,2,3,4
646.3	0,1,3
646.4 - 646.6	0,1,2,3,4
646.7	0,1,3

Categories and Subcategories	Fifth Digits
646.8	0,1,2,3,4
646.9	0,1,3
647 - 648	0,1,2,3,4
651 - 653	0,1,3
654.0 and 654.1	0,1,2,3,4
654.2	0,1,3
654.3 - 654.9	0,1,2,3,4
655 - 659	0,1,3
660 - 663	0,1,3
664	0,1,4
665.0	0,1,3
665.1	0,1
665.2	0,2,4
665.3 - 665.6	0,1,4
665.7	0,1,2,4
665.8 and 665.9	0,1,2,3,4
666 - 667	0,2,4
668	0,1,2,3,4
669.0 - 669.2	0,1,2,3,4
669.3	0,2,4
669.4	0,1,2,3,4
669.5 - 669.7	0,1
669.8 - 669.9	0,1,2,3,4
670	0,2,4
671.0 - 671.2	0,1,2,3,4
671.3	0,1,3

Categories and Subcategories	Fifth Digits
671.4	0,2,4
671.5 - 671.9	0,1,2,3,4
672	0,2,4
673	0,1,2,3,4
674.0	0,1,2,3,4
674.1 - 674.9	0,2,4
675 - 676	0,1,2,3,4

12. SKIN AND SUBCUTANEOUS TISSUE

681.0	0,1,2
681.1	0,1
686.0	0,1,9
690.1	0,1,2,8
692.7	0,1,2,3,4,5,9
692.8	1,2,3,9
694.6	0,1
695.8	1,9
702.1	1,9
704.0	0,1,2,9
705.8	1,2,3,9
707.1	0,1,2,3,4,5,9
709.0	0,1,9

13. MUSCULOSKELETAL SYSTEM

711 - 712	0,1,2,3,4,5,6,7,8,9
714.3	0,1,2,3

Categories and Subcategories	Fifth Digits
714.8	1,9
715.0	0,4,9
715.1 - 715.3	0,1,2,3,4,5,6,7,8
715.8	0,9
715.9	0,1,2,3,4,5,6,7,8
716.0 - 716.5	0,1,2,3,4,5,6,7,8,9
716.6	0,1,2,3,4,5,6,7,8
716.8 - 716.9	0,1,2,3,4,5,6,7,8,9
717.4	0,1,2,3,9
717.8	1,2,3,4,5,9
718.0 and 718.1	0,1,2,3,4,5,7,8,9
718.2 - 718.5	0,1,2,3,4,5,6,7,8,9
718.6	0,5
718.8	0,1,2,3,4,5,6,7,8,9
718.9	0,1,2,3,4,5,7,8,9
719.0 - 719.6	0,1,2,3,4,5,6,7,8,9
719.7	0,5,6,7,8,9
719.8 and 719.9	0,1,2,3,4,5,6,7,8,9
720.8	1,9
721.4	1,2
721.9	0,1
722.1	0,1
722.3	0,1,2,9
722.5	1,2
722.7 - 722.9	0,1,2,3
724.0	0,1,2,9

Categories and Subcategories	Fifth Digits
724.7	0,1,9
726.1	0,1,2,9
726.3	0,1,2,3,9
726.6	0,1,2,3,4,5,9
726.7	0,1,2,3,9
726.9	0,1
727.0	0,1,2,3,4,5,6,9
727.4	0,1,2,3,9
727.5	0,1,9
727.6	0,1,2,3,4,5,6,7,8,9
727.8	1,2,3,9
728.1	0,1,2,3,9
728.7	1,9
728.8	1,2,3,4,5,6,9
729.3	0,1,9
729.8	1,2,9
730	0,1,2,3,4,5,6,7,8,9
733.0	0,1,2,3,9
733.1	0,1,2,3,4,5,6,9
733.2	0,1,2,9
733.4	0,1,2,3,4,9
733.8	1,2
733.9	0,1,2,9
736.0	0,1,2,3,4,5,6,7,9
736.2 and 736.3	0,1,2,9
736.4	1,2

Categories and Subcategories	Fifth Digits
736.7	0,1,2,3,4,5,6,9
736.8	1,9
737.1 and 737.2	0,1,2,9
737.3	0,1,2,3,4,9
737.4	0,1,2,3
738.1	0,1,2,9

14. CONGENITAL ANOMALIES

741	0,1,2,3
742.5	1,3,9
743.0	0,3,6
743.1 and 743.2	0,1,2
743.3	0,1,2,3,4,5,6,7,9
743.4 and 743.5	1,2,3,4,5,6,7,8,9
743.6	1,2,3,4,5,6,9
744.0	0,1,2,3,4,5,9
744.2	1,2,3,4,9
744.4	1,2,3,6,7,9
744.8	1,2,3,4,9
745.1	0,1,2,9
745.6	0,1,9
746.0	0,1,2,9
746.8	1,2,3,4,5,6,7,9
747.1	0,1
747.2	0,1,2,9
747.4	0,1,2,9

Categories and Subcategories	Fifth Digits
747.6	0,1,2,3,4,9
747.8	1,2,9
748.6	0,1,9
749.0 and 749.1	0,1,2,3,4
749.2	0,1,2,3,4,5
750.1	0,1,2,3,5,6,9
750.2	1,2,3,4,5,6,7,9
751.6	0,1,2,9
752.1	0,1,9
752.4	0,1,2,9
752.5	1,2
752.6	1,2,3,4,5,9
753.1	0,1,2,3,4,5,6,7,9
753.2	0,1,2,3,9
754.3	0,1,2,3,5
754.4	0,1,2,3,4
754.5	0,1,2,3,9
754.6	0,1,2,9
754.7	0,1,9
754.8	1,2,9
755.0	0,1,2
755.1	0,1,2,3,4
755.2 and 755.3	0,1,2,3,4,5,6,7,8,9
755.5	0,1,2,3,4,5,6,7,8,9
755.6	0,1,2,3,4,5,6,7,9
756.1	0,1,2,3,4,5,6,7,9

Categories and Subcategories	Fifth Digits
756.5	0,1,2,3,4,5,6,9
756.7	0,1,9
756.8	1,2,3,9
757.3	1,2,3,9
758.8	1,9
759.8	1,2,3,9

15. CONDITIONS IN THE PERINATAL PERIOD

760.7	0,1,2,3,4,5,6,9
763.8	1,2,3,9
764 - 765	0,1,2,3,4,5,6,7,8,9
774.3	0,1,9

16. SYMPTOMS, SIGNS AND ILL-DEFINED CONDITIONS

780.0	1,2,3,9
780.3	1,9
780.5	0,1,2,3,4,5,6,7,9
780.7	1,9
781.9	1,2,9
782.6	1,2
783.2	1,2
783.4	0,1,2,3
784.4	0,1,9
784.6	0,1,9
785.5	0,1,9
786.0	0,1,2,3,4,5,6,7,9

Categories and Subcategories	Fifth Digits
786.5	0,1,2,9
787.0	1,2,3
787.9	1,9
788.2	0,1,9
788.3	0,1,2,3,4,5,6,7,9
788.4	1,2,3
788.6	1,2,9
789.0	0,1,2,3,4,5,6,7,9
789.3 and 789.4	0,1,2,3,4,5,6,7,9
789.6	0,1,2,3,4,5,6,7,9
790.0	1,9
790.9	1,2,3,4,9
794.0	0,1,2,9
794.1	0,1,2,3,4,5,6,7,9
794.3	0,1,9
795.7	1,9

14. INJURY AND POISONING

800 - 801	0,1,2,3,4,5,6,9
802.2 and 802.3	0,1,2,3,4,5,6,7,8,9
803 - 804	0,1,2,3,4,5,6,9
805.0 and 805.1	0,1,2,3,4,5,6,7,8
806.0 - 806.3	0,1,2,3,4,5,6,7,8,9
806.6 and 806.7	0,1,2,9
807.0 and 807.1	0,1,2,3,4,5,6,7,8,9
808.4 and 808.5	1,2,3,9

Categories and Subcategories	Fifth Digits
810	0,1,2,3
811	0,1,2,3,9
812.0 and 812.1	0,1,2,3,9
812.2 and 812.3	0,1
812.4 and 812.5	0,1,2,3,4,9
813.0 and 813.1	0,1,2,3,4,5,6,7,8
813.2 and 813.3	0,1,2,3
813.4 and 813.5	0,1,2,3,4
813.8 and 813.9	0,1,2,3
814	0,1,2,3,4,5,6,7,8,9
815	0,1,2,3,4,9
816	0,1,2,3
820.0 and 820.1	0,1,2,3,9
820.2 and 820.3	0,1,2
821.0 and 821.1	0,1
821.2 and 821.3	0,1,2,3,9
823	0,1,2
825.2 and 825.3	0,1,2,3,4,5,9
831	0,1,2,3,4,9
832	0,1,2,3,4,9
833	0,1,2,3,4,5,9
834	0,1,2
835	0,1,2,3
836.5 and 836.6	0,1,2,3,4,9
838	0,1,2,3,4,5,6,9
839.0 and 839.1	0,1,2,3,4,5,6,7,8

Categories and Subcategories	Fifth Digits
839.2 and 839.3	0,1
839.4 and 839.5	0,1,2,9
839.6 and 839.7	1,9
842.0	0,1,2,9
842.1	0,1,2,3,9
845.0 and 845.1	0,1,2,3,9
848.4	0,1,2,9
851 - 854	0,1,2,3,4,5,6,9
861.0 and 861.1	0,1,2,3
861.2 and 861.3	0,1,2
862.2 and 862.3	1,2,9
863.2 and 863.3	0,1,9
863.4 and 863.5	0,1,2,3,4,5,6,9
863.8 and 863.9	0,1,2,3,4,5,9
864	0,1,2,3,4,5,9
865	0,1,2,3,4,9
866	0,1,2,3
868	0,1,2,3,4,9
872.0 and 872.1	0,1,2
872.6 and 872.7	1,2,3,4,9
873.2 and 873.3	0,1,2,3,9
873.4 and 873.5	0,1,2,3,4,9
873.6 and 873.7	0,1,2,3,4,5,9
874.0 and 874.1	0,1,2
880	0,1,2,3,9
881	0,1,2

Categories and Subcategories	Fifth Digits
900.0	0,1,2,3
900.8	1,2,9
901.4	0,1,2
901.8	1,2,3,9
902.1	0,1,9
902.2	0,1,2,3,4,5,6,7,9
902.3	1,2,3,4,9
902.4	0,1,2,9
902.5	0,1,2,3,4,5,6,9
902.8	1,2,7,9
903.0	0,1,2
904.4	0,1,2
904.5	0,1,2,3,4
922.3	1,2,3
923.0	0,1,2,3,9
923.1 and 923.2	0,1
924.0 - 924.2	0,1
926.1	1,2,9
927.0	0,1,2,3,9
927.1 and 927.2	0,1
928.0 - 928.2	0,1
941	0,1,2,3,4,5,6,7,8,9
942	0,1,2,3,4,5,9
943	0,1,2,3,4,5,6,9
944	0,1,2,3,4,5,6,7,8
945	0,1,2,3,4,5,6,9

Categories and Subcategories	Fifth Digits
948.0	0
948.1	0,1
948.2	0,1,2
948.3	0,1,2,3
948.4	0,1,2,3,4
948.5	0,1,2,3,4,5
948.6	0,1,2,3,4,5,6
948.7	0,1,2,3,4,5,6,7
948.8	0,1,2,3,4,5,6,7,8
948.9	0,1,2,3,4,5,6,7,8,9
952.0 and 952.1	0,1,2,3,4,5,6,7,8,9
959.0	1,9
965.0	0,1,2,9
965.6	1,9
989.8	1,2,3,4,9
995.5	0,1,2,3,4,5,9
995.6	0,1,2,3,4,5,6,7,8,9
995.8	0,1,2,3,4,5,6,9
996.0	0,1,2,3,4,9
996.3	0,1,2,9
996.5	1,2,3,4,5,6,9
996.6	0,1,2,3,4,5,6,7,8,9
996.7	0,1,2,3,4,5,6,7,8,9
996.8	0,1,2,3,4,5,6,7,9
996.9	0,1,2,3,4,5,6,9
997.0	0,1,2,9

Categories and Subcategories	Fifth Digits
997.6	0,1,2,9
997.9	1,9
998.1	1,2,3
998.5	1,9
998.8	1,2,3,9

15. V CODES

Categories and Subcategories	Fifth Digits
V02.5	1,2,9
V02.6	0,1,2,9
V03.8	1,2,9
V07.3	1,9
V09.7-V09.9	0,1
V10.0	0,1,2,3,4,5,6,7,9
V10.1	1,2
V10.2	0,1,2,9
V10.4	0,1,2,3,4,5,6,7,8,9
V10.5	0,1,2,9
V10.6	0,1,2,3,9
V10.7	1,2,9
V10.8	1,2,3,4,5,6,7,8,9
V12.0	0,1,2,3,9
V12.4	0,1,9
V12.5	0,1,2,9
V12.7	0,1,2,9
V13.0	0,1,9
V13.6	1,9
V15.0	1,2,3,4,5,6,7,8,9

Categories and Subcategories	Fifth Digits
V15.4	1,2,9
V15.8	1,2,4,5,6,9
V16.4	0,1,2,3,9
V16.5	1,9
V18.6	1,9
V21.3	0,1,2,3,4,5
V23.8	1,2,3,4,9
V25.0	1,2,9
V25.4	0,1,2,3,9
V26.2	1,2,9
V26.5	1,2
V30 - V39 (with .0 fourth digit only)	0,1
V42.8	1,2,3,4,9
V43.6	0,1,2,3,4,5,6,9
V43.8	1,2,3,9
V44.5	0,1,2,9
V45.0	0,1,2,9
V45.5	1,2,9
V45.6	1,9
V45.7	1,2,3,4,5,6,7,8,9
V45.8	1,2,3,9
V49.6	0,1,2,3,4,5,6,7
V49.7	0,1,2,3,4,5,6,7
V49.8	1,9
V50.4	1,2,9
V53.0	1,2,9

Categories and Subcategories	Fifth Digits
V53.3	1,2,9
V56.3	1,2
V57.2	1,2
V57.8	1,9
V58.4	1,9
V58.6	1,2,9
V58.8	1,2,3,9
V59.0	1,2,9
V61.1	0,1,2
V61.2	0,1,2,9
V61.4	1,9
V62.8	1,2,3,9
V65.4	0,1,2,3,4,5,9
V67.0	0,1,9
V67.5	1,9
V68.8	1,9
V71.0	1,2,9
V71.8	1,9
V72.8	1,2,3,4,5
V73.8 and V73.9	8,9
V76.1	0,1,2,9
V76.4	1,2,3,4,5,6,7,9
V76.5	0,1,2
V76.8	1,9
V77.9	1,9
V82.8	1,9

APPENDIX D

THE 100 MOST COMMON DIAGNOSES

The following alphabetical list represents the 100 most commonly used ICD-9-CM codes. Codes followed by a single asterisk "*" require either a 4th *or* 5th digit for completion, depending on the code. (For example, if there is already a 4th digit, the single asterisk means a 5th digit is required.) Codes followed by a double asterisk "**" require both the 4th *and* 5th digit for completion.

Abdominal pain	789.0*
Acne rosacea	695.3
Acne vulgaris	706.1
Actinic keratosis	702.0
Allergic rhinitis	477.9
Amenorrhea	626.0
Anemia	281.9
Angina pectoris	413.*
ASHD (arteriosclerotic heart disease)	414.0*
Arthritis (osteo)	715.**
Arrhythmia	427.*
Asthma	493.**
Atherosclerosis	440.*
Back pain (NOS)	724.5
Bronchial asthma (NOS)	493.9*
Bronchitis, acute	496
Bronchitis, chronic	491.*
Bursitis (NOS)	727.3
Carpel tunnel syndrome	354.0
Cervicalgia/Pain in neck	723.1
Cesarean section	669.7*
Cervicitis	616.0
Chest pain	786.5*
Cholecystitis	575.*
CHF (congestive heart failure)	428.0
CVA (cerebrovascular disease)	436
Cyst, sebaceous	706.2

Cystic breast disease	610.1
Cystitis	595.*
Cystocele	618.0
Degenerative disc disease (NOS)	722.6
Delivery (Normal)	650
Dermatitis (NOS)	692.9
Diabetes Mellitus	250.**
Diverticulitis	562.1*
Dyshidrosis	705.81
Dysmenorrhea	625.3
Eczema (NOS)	692.9
Emphysema	492.*
Endometriosis	617.*
Fever (NOS)	780.6
Folliculitis	704.8
Gastroenteritis	558.*
Headache	784.0
Hemorrhoids	455.*
Hernia, inguinal	550.**
Herpes simplex	054.*
Herpes zoster (NOS)	053.9
Hypertension	401.*
Hypoglycemia	251.2
Immunization/vaccination	V03-V06.*
Influenza	487.*
Irritable bowel syndrome	564.1
Knee derangement	717.*
Lump in breast	611.72
Medical exam	V70.*
Menopausal syndrome	627.2
Menorrhagia	626.2
Mitral valve disease	394.*
Moniliasis/candidiasis	112.*
Muscle spasms	728.85
Myocardial infarction	410.**
Nasopharyngitis	460
Nephritis (acute)	580.*
Nephritis (chronic)	582.*
Nerve root irritation (neck)	353.2

Nerve root irritation (back)	724.4
Nevus	448.1
Obesity	278.0*
Onychomycosis	110.1
Otitis externa	380.1*
Otitis media	381.**
Pharyngitis	462
Pityriasis rosea	696.3
Pneumonia	486
Polymenorrhea	626.2
Post partum care	V24.2
Psoriasis (NOS)	696.1
Refractive errors	367.*
Scabies	133.0
Scoliosis	737.3*
Seborrheic dermatitis	690.1*
Sinusitis	461.*
Skin tags	701.9
Tachycardia	785.0
Thoracic outlet syndrome	353.0
Tinea cruris	110.3
Tinea corporis	110.5
Tinea pedis	110.4
Tinea versicolor	111.0
Tonsillitis, acute	463
Trichomoniasis	131.*
URI (upper respiratory infection)	465.*
UTI (urinary tract infection)	599.0
Vaginitis	616.10
Verruca	078.1*
Vertigo (NOS)	780.4
Viremia	790.8
Well-Baby Care	V20.2

INDEX